W9-CDH-289

The Business of Massage

DISCLAIMER

This book is designed to provide information in regard to the subject matter covered. It is sold with the understanding that the publisher and author are not engaged in rendering legal, accounting or other professional services. If legal or other expert assistance is required, the services of a competent professional should be sought.

It is not the purpose of this manual to reprint all the information that is otherwise available to the author and/or publisher, but to complement, amplify and supplement other texts. You are urged to read all the available material, learn as much as possible about massage and to tailor the information to your individual needs.

Every effort has been made to make this book as complete and as accurate as possible. However, there may be mistakes both typographical and in content. Therefore, this text should be used only as a general guide and not as the ultimate source for information on building a massage practice.

The purpose of this book is to educate and entertain. The author/publisher shall have neither liability nor responsibility to any person or entity with respect to any loss or damage caused, or alleged to be caused, directly or indirectly by the information contained therein.

The Business of Massage

A Manual for Students and Professionals

by Maryann Capó
Licensed Massage Therapist

10 9 8 7 6 5 4 3 2 1

Copyright © 1992 by Maryann Capó
First Printing 1992
Printed in the United States of America

ISBN 0-9631691-3-0 Softcover

What experienced health professionals are saying about

The Business of Massage
A Manual for Students and Professionals

"I could truly say (and I'm in this business 37 years) that this book was fascinating, and I wanted to go back repeatedly to recheck the helpful and honestly caring hints. For the new massage therapist this book is a great reference source. For those of us who are contented long-timers, who may have skimped on creativity in our professional and business approach, this book is an invitation to revitalize! Thanks for a gem!"

—ELIZABETH POST, Board Member
New York State Society of
Medical Massage Therapists

"This book tells you everything you need to know to start your massage practice... and keep it going. The information is bountiful — have a feast."

—ROCHELLE DONNINO
Licensed Massage Therapist

"A person who pursues a career in massage has certain altruistic aims — a desire to help others, a devotion to those in need, a giving, sharing quality. These attributes, together with well-developed technical skills, are part of what one needs to be a successful therapist. The third element in the success equation is business experience.

"Maryann Capó has chronicled her experience as a professional massage therapist to help the new and inexperienced practitioner survive in the business world. She offers practical advice on every facet of developing a practice, from understanding your own special attributes, how and where to set up a practice, to how to acquire new patients. Her procedures are clearly explained, are practical and ethical, and can assist any therapist in making their practice a prosperous business."

—DR. ROBERT BORZONE, Chiropractor
Dean of Western Sciences of the
New Center for Wholistic Health,
Education and Research

DEDICATED

**to all those fledgling professionals
who have a dream...**

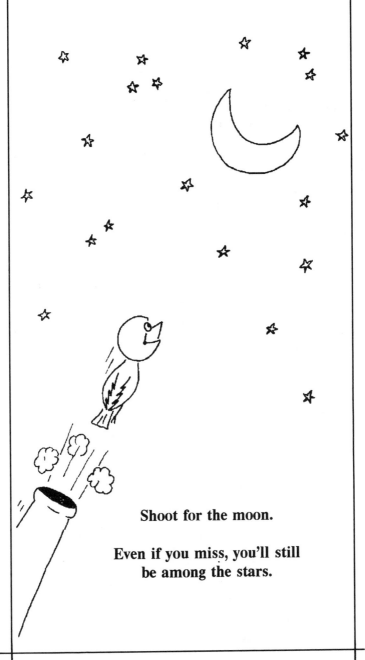

Shoot for the moon.

Even if you miss, you'll still
be among the stars.

Acknowledgments

- To my daughter-in-law Nancy, who took my ideas and gave them substance with her clever illustrations,

- To my son James, whose computer skills and business acumen brought life to my dream,

- To my granddaughter Michal Lisa, who modeled for her mother,

- To her little sister Jacqueline Lee, who was willing to share her mother with a drawing board,

- To my friend Lorraine LoMonaco, who kept encouraging me to stop talking and to take that first step,

I can only say "Thank You" for believing in me and for supporting me. Without you, this book would still be a figment of my very active imagination.

Illustrations by Nancy Capó

Foreword

by Harold Packman

Past President of the
New York State Society of Medical Massage Therapists
Author of
ICE THERAPY—UNDERSTANDING ITS APPLICATION

Perhaps the greatest advantage in being a Licensed Massage Therapist for 27 years, is the one-to-one professional relationship I have had, and still have, with my clientele and patients. I have had the opportunity over the years to see firsthand what makes for a successful practice; and I can tell you that for all of the schooling, for all of the training, for all of the skills needed to make a successful Massage Therapist, there are two major ingredients that finalize the success of any treatment given to the public. These two ingredients are: enthusiasm and attitude. I can admit to my own practice being solidly based on these wonderful keystones.

Over the years I have seen the general public reshaping its thinking about our healing profession, because of education, skill, and yes, our enthusiasm and attitude. Massage offers people more benefit to their individual lifestyles than just receiving a "rub down," and once we prove this to people, then a "truth" has been realized.

"Harold, I canceled $2,700 worth of surgery this morning to keep my massage appointment with you; that's how I feel about Massage Therapy," said one of my clients, an OB-GYN who received massage twice weekly. The spouse of a stroke patient once told me, "My husband had not slept eight hours in a month, until you came into his life."

Maryann Capó has obviously worked diligently through the various preparations, the details, the equipment, the ambiance necessary for the Massage Therapist to be able to concentrate his or her skills on the practice at hand. What will also benefit the client and patient is the *enthusiasm* and *attitude* coming from the therapist.

Maryann has truly brought her knowledge, her experience, her vibrancy, her warmth, *and* her enthusiasm and attitude, throughout the pages of her book. Attitude *is* a "two-way street" — what you put out is what you get back.

Harold Packman
"The Ice Man"
December, 1991

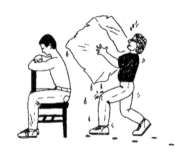

Author's Preface

Have you ever thought about the convoluted path you've traveled on the journey toward your life's goal? How the twists and turns have brought you to this spot at this time?

As a teenager I had no defined work goal. I idolized my brother who was a bomber pilot during World War II and I wanted to fly like he did. Back in those "ancient" times, however, women did not *fly* planes, they were flight attendants. And in those hazardous early days, the attendants were required to be nurses... not for me, thank you.

Many years later I did get to take power flight and sailplane lessons, and even went for a thrilling ride in a hot air balloon... piloted by a retired Air Force Colonel!

It is ironic that in my youth I had no inclination for medicine, yet here I am in this most exciting branch of the healing professions. But before I became a massage therapist I was a Sales Rep—which is another way of saying I lived in my car.

I became an expressway maniac, bucking rush hour traffic, summer road construction, and freezing snow and ice in the winter. I was such a mass of tension I was faced with the choice of finding a therapist to work out my spasmed muscles, or quitting my job.

Well, I did both. I started studying massage, became a therapist, and loved it so much that I left my salaried position and plunged into my new career at the age of 59.

Establishing a viable practice without capital or experience was no picnic. I had a lot to learn, with no mentor to guide me. There were plenty of frustrations, time consuming false starts and numerous costly errors to overcome before I felt I was finally on the right track.

This book has been written in hopes that it will save you valuable time and effort. I hope it will inspire you and encourage you to keep trying... Cicero said it best, "The greater the difficulty, the greater the glory."

Maryann Capo
Lake Ronkonkoma, NY
December 16, 1991

Table of Contents

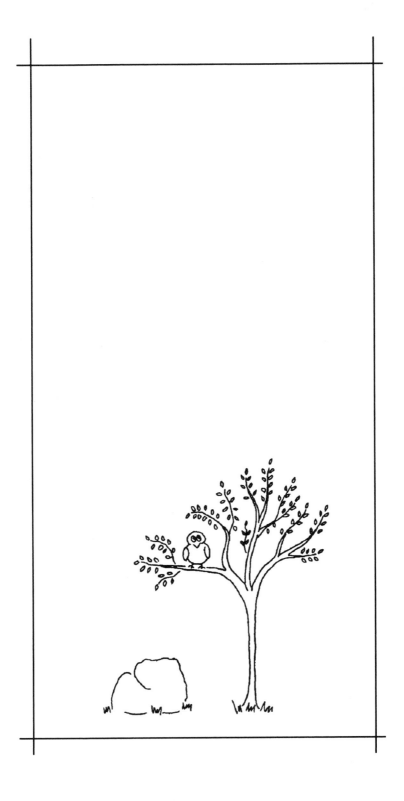

PART ONE

Grow Your Business

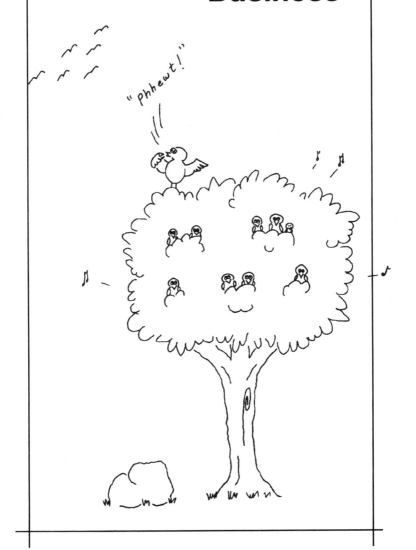

The world stands aside to let anyone pass who knows where he is going.

--Author unknown

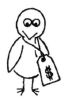

Your Most Important Asset

"I have my license, so... *what do I do NOW?"*

Good question, you say. Do you:
- a) order business cards
- b) set up office
- c) organize client files
- d) none of the above
- e) all of the above

The answer is D. Are you surprised? And well you should be. After all, isn't this book about your massage business? But acquiring technical skills does not necessarily guarantee you success. Hanging out your shingle will not make people beat a path to your door.

The days of the family physician who came to your house when you were ill are gone, and with him went his caring bedside manner. How often have you heard, "I went to the doctor and I couldn't understand a word he said", or, "I went for some physical therapy and it didn't help — all they did was attach some machines to me and then left me alone in the room."

Your most important asset is YOU. Your character traits, your perspectives, your *personality*. Do you listen to what your client *isn't* saying? Can you empathize with the the emotional pain your clients may be experiencing? Are you secure enough within yourself to forget who *you* are and concentrate on who *they* are and what *their* needs are?

The following guidelines will help you focus on the important points that will act as your lighthouse in the turbulent sea of life.

1. Proportion. Maintain a sense of perspective and proportion in all your endeavors. What appears to be the most monumental obstacle, the most devastating setback when you are standing beside it, becomes less and less important as you distance yourself from it. Don't let what happened yesterday inhibit what *is* happening today or *will* happen tomorrow. The mind is like a magnifying glass: it exaggerates. What you are looking at now may not be as big a deal as you think it is.

2. Perseverance. Perseverance is POWER. Don't give up!!! Go the distance and give it everything you've got. Like Rome, your career won't be built in a day. Remember Thomas Edison's pearl of wisdom: "Genius is 1% inspiration and 99% perspiration." Hang on through the rough seas. Your reward will be a following wind and smooth sailing.

3. Preparation. Preparation gives you *control* over a situation. It gives you the strength to follow through, so practice, practice, practice. The road to success is not on the Indianapolis Raceway. It is more like driving slowly along a curving, twisting, treacherous dirt road.

Be prepared for the unexpected while keeping a firm, solid grip on the wheel.

4. Focus. Concentrate all your energies on the task at hand. You have at your disposal the two most marvelously devised and efficient machines ever created: The human body, and the human mind. They can work wonders. They can move mountains. Focus every particle of your being on your goal. Like a runner straining toward the finish line, surge ahead and never look back!

5. Expertise. Become an expert. Hone your skill; learn as much about it as you can. Nothing can boost your confidence or increase your practice faster than knowing you are the best you can be. From knowledge comes authority. From authority comes power.

6. Responsibility. *Take* responsibility and people will *give* you responsibility. Take responsibility for the health and well-being of yourself and your clients. Take responsibility for the quality of your work. Take responsibility and you will take the lead. Be the kind of person people can trust and believe in. It will pay off.

7. Self-Awareness. Know what you can do; know what you can't do. Know when to listen to yourself; know when to seek advice. Know when to conserve energy; know when to expend it. Know when to push ahead; know when to retreat. Know what you want to achieve—and know the pleasure of getting it!

8. Image. Your demeanor — the way you look, the way you act, the way you express yourself—is your business card... it's what you leave behind. It's how people remember you. *Act* self-confident and you will *be* self-confident. The image you have of yourself is the image you project to others. Your mind is a perfect computer, and *you* are the programmer. What you put into the computer is what you'll get back. Isn't that a marvelous concept? So start pressing those keys. Just be sure you press the right ones!

9. Spirit. Listen to your hopes, your dreams, your desires. Follow where they lead. If you don't enjoy what you're doing, there's no point in wasting time doing it... you'll never be a success at it. Take risks, explore new possibilities, revive your spirit of enthusiasm, awaken your spirit of adventure. Who knows what's around the next corner or over the next hill. The thrill of finding out will keep the sparkle in your eye and anticipation in your step.

10. Seed. Remember that the embryo of self-confidence is within you. Exercise it, nurture it, delight in it—then anything can happen...

BELIEVE IT!

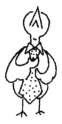

Your Professional Image: Is Dressing for Success A Myth or Reality?

Once upon a time, massage was found in two main localities — the "gym" and the "parlour."

In the gym, a big brawny masseur with bulging muscles stressing the constraints of his tank top, and with sweat pouring off his brow, pummeled and pounded the athlete on his table. If the athlete won his event, the masseur was a success and in demand.

In the parlour, a masseuse dressed in black lace stockings, skin tight revealing top and short skirt, lathered her client in oil and proceeded to give him an enticing "rub" which had little to do with a therapeutic toning of stressed muscles. If her dress and her demeanor succeeded in feeding her "John's" fantasy and resulted in a nice tip, she had dressed for success.

In a medical or clinical setting where the treatment of injuries is the concern of the therapist, then the comforting professional look of whites is appropriate.

23

In my office, I choose to appear conservative yet friendly. I wear a nice pair of white pants (not sweats), with a T-shirt (not a tank top), and a *good* pair of flat sneaker-type shoes. I discovered dove-grey shoes accidentally when the salesperson brought them out instead of the whites I had asked for. Now they are my favorites. My T-shirts carry the slogan, "It's Great To Be Kneaded," or "Massage Therapists Feel Kneaded." Don't forget... it pays to advertise!

On-site body therapy is pushing to enter the main-stream. We now have another chance to "Dress for Success." Are tank tops and sweatpants, or black lace and tight tops, or even medicinal whites, appropriate in this setting? I, for one, think not. A therapist wishing to enter a business office needs to dress in business attire in order to blend in with the surroundings, and be as non-disruptive of office routine as possible. But here again, care needs to be taken concerning what consti-tutes "business attire." Spike-heeled sandles and low cut dresses have no place here. Money for a new wardrobe needn't be a problem — a nice skirt or slacks with a few pretty mix-and-match blouses and low-heeled shoes can become a very serviceable "uniform." For the gentle-men, a pair of dark pants with a light colored polo shirt can fit the bill just as well.

Is dressing for success a reality? I say yes. If we want to change the way the world sees us, we need to change the way *we* see us.

Setting Up
Your Office

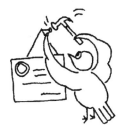

Your basic tools include the massage table and the space that surrounds it, your oils, and other necessities.

Your Table

The purchase of the major tool of your trade, the massage table, requires thought and consideration before committing large sums of money to its acquisition.

Will you be working in a spa? They may provide a table. Do you plan on doing mostly out-calls? A lighter table may be preferable.

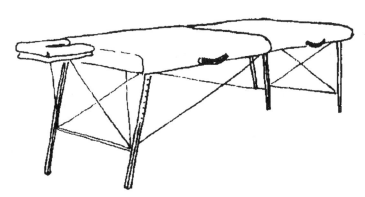

A light, portable table, like this one from Ultra-Light, Inc., 16 Dickerson Ave., Toms River, NJ 08753 (1-800-999-1971), is essential for a massage therapist doing lots of out-calls.

Is the space limited? You will need to have a table with a shelf underneath to store sheets and towels.

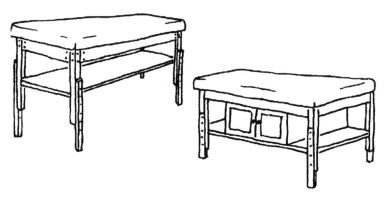

Tables with shelves come in a variety of styles. These attractive designs are from Living Earth Crafts®.

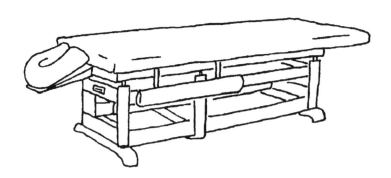

Having a table that allows for on-command height adjustment is valuable for the therapist with clients of many different sizes and builds. This table is by Stacy-Built Systems.

Do you anticipate clients of such different sizes as to require on-command height control of your table? Stacy-Built Systems (P.O. Box 1032, Clinton, NC 28328), among others, sells some.

Will you be doing on-site chair massage? You will need a High-Touch Massage Chair, and/or a Massage Mate Face Cradle.

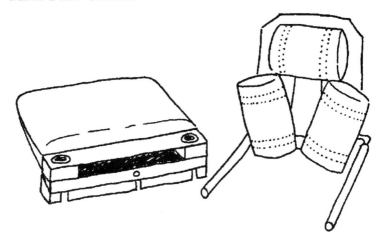

The light, easily portable Massage-Mate Face Cradle attaches quickly to the edge of a table or desk for go-anywhere chair massage.

Length and width, as well as durability, are also major considerations. A professional massage table is usually six feet by two feet and should be adjustable to your height. If the table is too low, you will find *yourself* in need of a massage. If it is too high, you lose the all-important leverage you need to be effective. For the average sized man or woman, 29 to 31 inches is the right height range.

A useful addition to your table is a set of side extenders. If you are a small person, do not buy a very wide table because you will have to stretch to reach across your client's back. If you find yourself with a muscle-builder type, or a 300-pound Goliath, the side extenders are very effective for handling the overflow.

A table with 2 1/2" double wrap foam provides luxurious comfort. An added nicety is a lamb's skin pad for more softness and table protection.

Speaking of coverings, I have an aversion to white sheets. They are cold. They stain. And they conjure up pictures of unpleasant hospital stays. I watch for "white" sales and buy colored, floral and striped *single* flannel sheets — I prefer these to fitted sheets (see the chapter on "Handitis"). I also go the extra expense of sheet towels which cover all but the very largest of my clients from head to toe.

With regard to those substantial clients — if you don't want to find yourself picking them up off the floor, be sure your table is sturdy enough to accommodate every precious pound of them... nor does a table that squeaks and groans allow for a very relaxing massage.

Physical Setting

Now it's time to set the stage. You are the star, and your client is the lead player. The main prop (your table) is in place. An ideal space which provides ample room to move around measures eight feet by 12 feet. Of course, you may not have the luxury of this much room in the beginning, and you *can* work in a smaller area, but

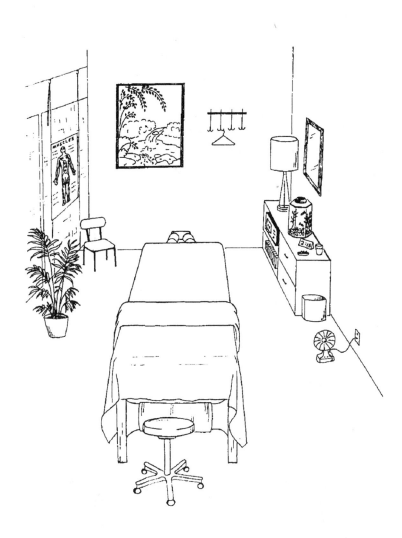

A fully outfitted work area, as described in this chapter, is both warm and comfortable for your clients, and easy for you to work in. This view is from the foot of the massage table.

why not set your sights high. After all, much of your working life will be spent here. If you are happy and comfortable, you can be sure your clients will pick up on that!

The next item to put in place is a side table large enough to hold a clock, a lamp, a cassette player with tapes, a small bottle of oil and a shallow dish to hold breath mints (more on this later). Hooks on the wall

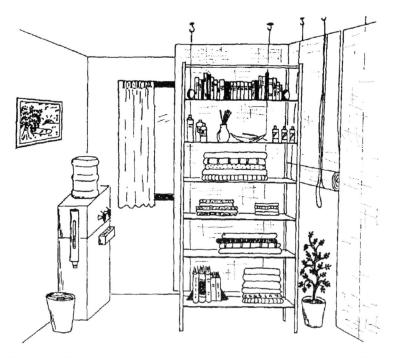

From the foot of the massage table, looking toward shelves holding sheets and towels, incense burner, oils and other supplies. Water cooler is on the left.

will hold your client's clothing and a mirror will allow for a final rearranging of hair and make-up. An eight inch portable fan on the floor can be moved around to allow you to regulate *your* fluctuating thermostat without cooling down your client's. Anatomical charts on the wall add a professional tone. Open shelves for clean sheets and towels... a hamper *under* the table for soiled linen... a chair for your client... a stool at the head of the table for you (and another near the foot of the table if you do reflexology)... a water cooler, and presto, your sanctuary is ready. The physical aspects are in place, and the "stage" is set.

Environment

Now it is time to consider the emotional setting—sight, sound, smell, touch.

With a clean, neat area, low lighting (heaven forbid you use overhead fluorescents!), the soothing sounds of an environmental tape, the smell of a scented candle or incense, the warmth of a flannel sheet and your caring touch now it's time to begin!

Oils and How Best to Use Them

Once you lay your hands on your client, do not break contact until the massage is over. How do you do this when you are ready to apply oil? I rest the back of my hand discreetly on my client's body, pour oil in my cupped hand, lay the bottle against a bolster (see Figure 6), rub my hands together to warm the oil, and apply to the area where I am working. I find the bolster a very

31

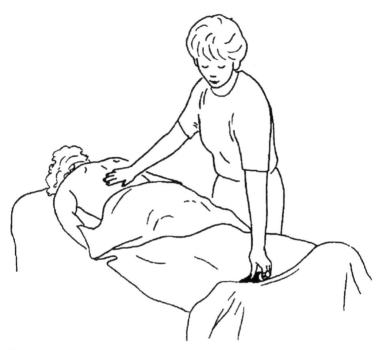

Resting your bottle of oil against a bolster placed under your client's knees (or ankles, if you're working on the back) gives you easy access without breaking touch during the massage.

convenient resting place which I can reach from anywhere around the table.

Speaking of **oils**—I have tried several types and brands and have settled on **Biotone** (3536 Adams Ave., San Diego, CA 92116) as my oil of choice. It is a light oil with a good balance between glide and firmness. It is especially effective during the summer months when my clients come in hot and sticky or when their tans begin to peel. There have been times when instead of dust balls under the massage table, I have had skin balls hanging off my fingers... yuk!

In the beginning, to keep costs down, I suggest using the unscented revitalizing oil if yours is a general practice. Some people are allergic to scents, so if you use unscented you are ahead of the game.

As your business progresses, you may want to keep an assortment of 4-oz. scented oils for a change of pace. Names such as Citrus, Coco-Almond, Lemon, Peach and Vanilla can really get the salivary glands flowing!

For the nature lover, there is Lavender, Wildflower or Woodsy Musk.

Clients will begin to express their preferences as you give them the opportunity to sample each fragrance. For a personalized touch, mark this information on their client card—your caring will make points, causing you to rise high in their estimation. Do the same with their musical preferences.

If your career turns toward sports massage or medical massage, there is a Therapeutic/Sports oil in an herbal blend. For those clients who do not like oils or are allergic to them, use the Massage Creme with arnica and ivy, or the Deep Tissue Massage Lotion.

No bees, no honey.

No work, no money.

--Avon

Where to Find

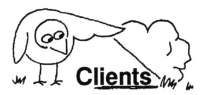

Before you begin record keeping, you need clients to keep track of. One of the first questions that comes up is, "Where do I find clients?" Next in importance is, "What do I charge?" Then when you start to build a following, the question becomes, "How do you handle men who come on to you?"— or for masseurs, "What do we do when women give a different meaning to the term therapeutic massage?" Most distressing of all is what to say to someone who calls looking for sexual favors?

All these questions will be answered. You will learn how to keep simple records; how to keep your client file; what to do to keep clients coming back; how to take care of yourself; how to handle different types of clients and suggestions on how to add to your income.

But first things first — finding your clients.

Expand from your Nucleus

Begin with the friends and relatives you worked on for free when you were a student. Make them the nucleus of your business. Send out announcement cards stating that you are open for business. They become your working capital. Tell them they are stockholders in your new company and that in order for them to receive dividends (discounts or reduced rates on their massages) your company must be profitable. Therefore, make them understand that you must charge. Make it a token fee, but ask them to pay something.

To sweeten the pot, tell them they will receive a 10% discount for every *paying* client they refer to you. Paying means they book and *keep* the appointment. Then you credit the person who referred them. I always ask how a person got my name, and mark the information on their Client Information card (see next chapter on KEEPING RECORDS). I also make a note on the card of the person doing the referring so that I will remember to give the discount the next time he or she comes in.

Advertise

It does pay to advertise, but use your money wisely. Advertising can be very expensive. I once (and only once) paid $900 for an ad in the Business to Business Yellow Pages. I received one inquiry for the whole year. Your major area newspaper may also be expensive. I have paid $490 for a one-shot deal, with very little return for my investment.

On the other hand, my one line listing in the regular telephone book Yellow Pages has been my best source for new clients.

In addition, I do very well with a small ad in my local Chamber of Commerce publication. I also submit articles, which I don't have to pay for — this is one way of establishing yourself as an "expert." In the ads I offer a 10% discount (everyone likes a bargain).

By this means I regularly add to my client file, and continue to keep in touch with them for future business. Each month I submit an article — on massage, reflexology, stress management — again with the 10% discount ad. I continue submitting articles so that people begin to look for my name. One of the first rules of advertising is consistency.

I also hand out reprints of these articles to new clients. This, again, helps establish me in their minds as an expert in my field.

The key with advertising is not how much money you spend doing it, but that the money is *wisely spent*. A small ad that is well-placed will do a lot more for you than some expensive ads will. And there are ways of "advertising" — getting your name known — that are free, and build a strong image as well. Like the articles. Also, if there is a Wholistic Health Directory in your area, it is a good idea to have yourself listed in it. You will be targeting people who are interested in health.

In the words of Stewart Britt, "Doing business without advertising is like winking in the dark — you know what you are doing, but nobody else does."

Contacts

Talk to everyone — your mechanic, your hairdresser, people standing in line with you. Leave your card under the tip you leave the waitress. Do you know how sore a busy waitress can be at the end of her day? Your pretty cards won't bring you business sitting on your desk — use them! Try writing a short message on the back — "Thanks — you're a super waitress. Stop by with this card some time and I'll give you a 10% discount on a massage."

Join community service organizations such as Kiwanis, Lion's, Rotary, Chamber of Commerce. These "old boy networks" are now accepting women as members, too. You will have access to mailing lists once you become a member. It will help you get into the mainstream of the business world, it will help to widen your circle of acquaintances with whom you can network, and it will help with referrals.

Join local business organizations. For female therapists, the National Association for Female Executives has local chapters which provide women with tools to achieve career success. And women's groups can be especially good for networking. Offer to Showcase one of their meetings. The meeting planners are always looking for interesting speakers to spice up the meeting.

Make Your Name Known

One of the cheapest and most effective ways to get your name before the public is through free publicity. Offer to give a talk at the Rotary Club, for instance, on Stress in the Workplace and the Benefits of Massage. Do a good job presenting and you will almost certainly gain new clients, and you will pave the way for other speaking engagements as well (see chapter 7 on ADDI-TIONAL INCOME).

After your free speech, send a press release to your local paper. If you can send a black and white photo with the release, you have an even better chance of making the headlines... and when you do, use the announcement as a flyer. A little horn-blowing never hurts!

When you write a press release, always include the words FOR IMMEDIATE RELEASE at the top, in all caps. The following are examples of how to write a press release:

FOR IMMEDIATE RELEASE

Maryann Capó, President of Ten Plus Ten, The Body & Sole Corp., was guest speaker at a recent Lindenhurst Kiwanis Club dinner.

Ms. Capó's audience-participation talk was on "Hug Therapy, the Happiest Path to Stress Management."

Contact: Maryann Capó
585-5691

The following press release appeared word-for-word in my local paper, under the photo I had enclosed with the copy. It had been titled, "Who's Who":

FOR IMMEDIATE RELEASE

Maryann Capó, President of Ten Plus Ten, The Body & Sole Corp., based in Lake Ronkonkoma, has been included in the 1989/1990 Who's Who of Woman Executives.

Ms. Capó's company offers "Work At Peak" programs, Surviving Stress Sensibly lectures, plus on-site 15-minute chair massage.

Contact: Maryann Capó
585-5691

The photo was run a column wide and four inches tall, plus the copy. Why pay for space advertising when you can get the exposure free, for the cost of a stamp and a photo?

Offer "Freebies"

Visit toning/tanning establishments and beauty/nail salons. Leave a card with the manager. Offer to give complimentary chair massage one day to introduce massage to the customers. Give a 10% discount on the next massage and book it on the spot. Build up the advantages to the manager: Customers have something to do while waiting; massage is another specialized service offered their clientele; massage is a tension reliever; chair massage doesn't require removal of clothing and there is no oil used which could destroy a new "do."

For giving you space to ply your trade, give the manager a free massage each week that you have clients booked. I know of a salon which is incorporating aromatherapy along with the chair massage.

Tap the Health Trade

Don't forget the health clubs and spas. The clubs usually ask you to rent the space and then you keep the fee charged to the customer — an iffy situation if the club is not active enough to supply you with enough clients to pay the rent and then have money for yourself. When I worked the fitness centers, I only paid the club when I had a customer. They would book the appointment, call me and I would give them part of the fee.

Michael J. Aronoff, a therapist working at the Body By Berle gym in Great Neck, NY, gets clients used to the idea of massage by offering a complimentary chair massage to any new client of the gym. Of course they like it, book regular body massage and begin to refer him to friends. He now has the best kind of a practice, one built on satisfied clients.

I have left my cards in the weight room at the local hotels, and with desk clerks. Several of the people referred from this source have become steady clients.

Leave your cards at health food stores, even your local delicatessen — anywhere there is high traffic volume. I left cards in a card holder on the counter (ask permission) with a small sign stating that I would give anyone who mentioned the deli when making an appointment a

10% discount. I also said I would give the employees of the deli a 10% discount — a win-win situation!

As I received clients from this source, I tacked a notice in the deli so the employees would know how many massages were credited to them. Super advertising because when people asked if I was good, the employees enthusiastically replied in the affirmative. Word of mouth is your best and cheapest form of advertising — encourage it however you can.

And don't forget the bulletin boards at the laundromats. You never know where or when a new client will come along.

Other Professionals

Of course, make the rounds of you local chiropractors, who can turn out to be a great source of referrals. Chiropractic and massage make a wonderful team. In fact, more and more chiropractors have a therapist on staff.

I have devised a "Letter of Medical Necessity" which I give to clients seeking medical reimbursement (see page 84). In this way the medical profession also becomes a member of the team as more people demand a substitute for drug therapy. The letter and my receipt for services rendered are submitted to the insurance company.

Not all insurance companies are recognizing massage therapy yet, but we are making in-roads. Eventually, as more and more physicians acknowledge the benefits to their patients, the insurance companies will also come around. I try not to accept assignment because I don't like to wait months for the insurance company to pay me — and when they do, it is only a small part of my fee. Rather, I prefer to give my client a discount when the situation warrants it. This makes for a win-win arrangement and we are both happy.

If you want to pursue this avenue more thoroughly, there are books on "How to Get Reimbursed" listed in the Appendix at the end of this book.

Explore Your Options

Recently I was asked to make a house call for a lady with scoliosis. I have limited my out-calls as my practice has grown, but I do go out for senior citizens who are infirm or who don't drive.

"Well," my caller replied, "we qualify on both counts."

As I give a discount for seniors, the lady gave her okay even though I charge more for an out-call. To help her even more, I gave her the discount coupon I had placed in the Chamber of Commerce publication — even though she hadn't seen it herself. Though I gave her two discounts (she was thrilled), I still made money myself. Win-win situation! She and her sister discovered that a bus goes right past my office so *both* of them are now coming to me.

A small discount in the beginning can pay off in the end. Appropriate generosity and extending human kindness are rewarding and satisfying emotionally *and* financially.

Speaking of seniors — you may want to consider the "Graying of America" and specialize. The older generation is becoming a major consumer of the service industry. It can be a very satisfying area to tap because you can provide them with a valuable, needed and appreciated service.

While aging muscles benefit greatly from therapeutic massage, often it is the personal attention, the *caring* touch, that is given to the isolated, infirm older person that is even more beneficial to them. The emotional care and sensitivity that is part of a good massage, that is shown to them as individuals, can restore some of the sense of personal value that is so often missing in their lives.

Yet many grandparents today are putting their younger relatives to shame... they have time, many have disposable funds, they are more vibrant, they take care of themselves and they want to enjoy what time is remaining to them. They have retired to adult communities — a one-spot-stop for you and your service. All these communities have a recreation room. Speak with the Recreation Director and ask to be put on the program as a guest speaker. Then put together a demo-lecture.

Let the residents know that you will be available to go to their room or to their condo where you will give them a full body massage, a chair massage, a reflexology treatment (all older people have sore feet!), or whatever else you want to offer. Don't forget to work in your discount program!

Another avenue to pursue is the Resort Hotels. The pay may be nominal, but the room and board plus the vacation spot itself could make up for the small salary.

Enterprising therapists are following the sun in a different way — they set up their chair or table at the beach. Others become part of fairs and charge $1 a minute for chair massage.

Out-Call Savvy.

General out-calls can become your specialty, though you need to be more careful than you would be for the senior market. Remember, you are going to a stranger's home at night. For a woman therapist, a good idea is to wear a wedding ring and tell you client that your husband expects you to call him when you arrive at your destination and again when you are ready to leave. A girlfriend, mother, neighbor, etc., can stand in for a non-existent "husband."

(When I have to work late at night at my office, especially in dark winter months, I enlist my girlfriend's aid. She calls when she knows I will be finishing up. Since my answering machine is always on, she leaves a message saying she is on her way over in 15 minutes so we can go for coffee).

Richard Cowan, a therapist licensed in both massage and physical therapy, makes house visits in New York City and Long Island. It has been his experience that it is not unusual for husbands to not approve of their wives being massaged by a male.

He recounted one situation where he had been massaging both the male and female members of the household. After several visits, the man decided to forego his treatments, but the woman continued with hers... and then it happened.

It was a windy, rainy night outside, but cozy and comfortable inside. The atmosphere was right for a massage — the lights were subdued and the music was soft and low. Suddenly Rich spotted movement out of the corner of his eye. As he turned to face the window, he saw a shadow reflected on the wet surface of the window sill. After checking with his client to be sure there was nothing that could cause this phenomenon (they were on the 13th floor of a New York building), he raised the windowshade. He jumped back in surprise, for there stood someone dressed all in black and dripping wet!

When Richard's client asked her husband later if anyone had been on their 13th floor terrace, he answered, "no one" and denied peeking in at them. Yet he was dressed in black and was all wet. The woman wanted to continue her sessions, but Rich would do so only if the man admitted to, and apologized for, watching them. Since neither declaration was forthcoming, Richard made the decision not to return.

Still, despite occasional problems like this, there are still a number of legitimate people who desire house-calls for the convenience, and not for sexual titillation.

We are such a stressed-out society that many people want to have a massage and then roll over and go to bed. For them, that is the only way to truly relax.

This can be a very lucrative business if handled prudently. The service business is on the upswing. Massage is being used as perks and bonuses, people feel that because they work so hard that they deserve to pamper themselves — but even more important, they realize that it is necessary for their health and the success of their job to be in good physical condition. Just be sure that you don't sell your time cheaply. Tack on an extra $15 to your normal fee. Remember you have to take into consideration your time going and coming, the time spent in massaging, gas and depreciation on your car.

I have two tables. One remains in my office, the other I keep in my car for the times I have out-calls. I am ready at a moment's notice and can get where I'm going with little stress on my part because I am always prepared. I have a tote bag packed with a sheet, towel, oil, client card and health questionnaire.

If you do transport your table for outcalls, save your back by using a sturdy luggage carrier — it is a great back saver. Some carrying cases have wheels already attached. Do whatever is necessary to prevent your own fatigue.

Volunteer at Sports Outings

I have volunteered my services at Golf Outings. I receive free publicity in the journal/program. Of course, while I am massaging, I ask the golfers to "sign in" with

47

their names and addresses. Presto! Another mailing list. I have gotten some very nice, regular clients this way.

After the event I write to everyone telling them I enjoyed meeting them, that I hoped they liked the massage and that it had helped improve their game. A month or so before the Holidays I send a letter suggesting chair massage as a bonus gift for their employees.

This is another example of how occasionally giving away something for free can work to your benefit in the long run.

Capitalize On the Moment

If you have an answering machine, make it work for you. During the holidays I jog people's memories by reminding them that gift certificates make a great gift for that someone who has everything.

One of my messages said, "Happy holidays! Maryann speaking. [Now here comes the pitch] — A massage gift is a gift of health for yourself or someone you care about." Then I ask them to leave their name and number so I can return the call. I pulled in an extra $2,000 on gift certificates alone!

Also, have a sign in your place of business stating that you have gift certificates available. Make it in eye-catching colors and enumerate the many occasions for a gift — the usual birthday, anniversary, Valentine's Day, Secretary's Day, Grandparents Day, as a Thank You, engagement or pre-wedding gift, or "Just Because."

And about Gift Certificates, even though you are not getting paid at the time of the treatment, go all out to surpass your best treatment techniques. When a prospective client walks in with a certificate, the "bait" is set — you "hook" him with your excellent treatment, and you reel him in when you follow up with Birthday, Christmas or "I was thinking of you" cards (see KEEPING IN TOUCH, later).

Free On-Site "Mini's"

A word about the new kid on the block — chair massage.

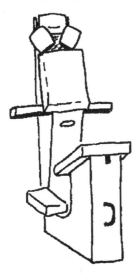

I use Living Earth Crafts Massage Mate. (See the diagram on page 27). It is extremely portable, comes with its own carrying case, and easily attaches to the edge of a table or desk. It goes anywhere, even on a plane since it is no larger than a tote bag. Now you can truly say, "Have hands, will travel!"

If you don't mind the extra weight, the High-Touch Massage Chair is a nice, compact, stand-alone unit. I used it when I first started going into corporations, but at 25.5 pounds I found it a little heavy for my weak back.

If you need a stand-alone unit for on-site chair massage, the High-Touch Massage Chair is well made and folds down to a compact box, but some may find it is a bit heavy.

So I keep my Massage Mate always in my car, available at a moment's notice. I am a member of the American Heart Association's Walking Club. We walk in the local mall, the inside perimeter of which measures one mile. Since I finish my four miles earlier than most everyone else, I set up my Massage Mate with a sign reading "Free Massage — compliments of Ten + Ten." I have flyers available offering a discount on a full hour massage. My business cards are also available and since my fellow walkers know me, they feel confident booking an appointment.

I "dot" each person with a Stressdot so they can see how the mini-massage starts reducing their stress right away. There is a Bonger on the table which draws quite a few questions. (See Part 7 on ADDED INCOME). People waiting in line for their massage start bongering themselves and prospective sales are in the making.

A word of advice: Always get permission from the mall to set up your little "concession stand." Don't step on any toes. Even though there is no exchange of money, the mall may object to your arbitrarily assuming you can do what you want on their property.

Shopping Malls

Malls could prove to be the sleeper of the century. Why not become a "Temporary Tenant"? Depending on the contract terms made between you and the mall management, you can become a permanent/temporary tenant for one week, a month, eight weeks during the holiday season, or a year.

Becoming a specialty leasing tenant can benefit both you and the mall developers. Successful temporary carts (generally supplied by the mall) and kiosk programs (permanent installations) not only fill empty space in mall corridors, but also provide an interesting mix of tenants.

What a perfect set-up for chair massage! Weary shoppers can stop by for a few minutes of TLC and then sally forth, refreshed and ready to continue their shopping. Husbands left to shift for themselves can find solace while waiting for the missus to reclaim them. You can set aside space to do reflexology to ease the pain of shoppers' feet.

Though mall corridor space can be expensive, what exposure you will have! Especially if you can afford a lease during the holiday season. Think of all the Gift Certificates you can sell and how many full body massages you can book. You have a group of vulnerable people — frazzled and hurting from shopping and frustrated because they can't find "the perfect gift" for that person who has everything.

Here is an excellent opportunity to put your teamwork skills to work. Get together with other therapists with whom you are compatible. You can set yourselves up as a partnership or you can work individually, sharing the expense of the space but keeping your own fees. Because the area must be manned during the mall hours, it would be advantageous to have more than one therapist on hand.

In order to provide the most service and to provide the opportunity for the most revenue, partner up with one or two chair massage therapists, reflexologists, Shiatsu and

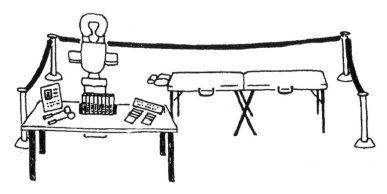

Set up in a mall corridor as part of a health fair, or as a temporary tenant. It can be lucrative at the right season, especially for Gift Certificate sales, and it provides great exposure.

Trager practitioners. You can share rental costs, and hours while exposing a large group of individuals to a variety of modalities.

Depending on how many will be working the space at any given time, an open area of about 5' x 7' would be a good starting point. The area could be roped off by four upright supports, connected with decorative roping. You can also provide more privacy by using low wooden partitions. Try making your "shop" as portable as possible so it can be easily moved from mall to mall.

You might want to make shelves to display whatever wholistic products you would like to offer for sale — another avenue of revenue. Be identifiable, be original, be creative. Set yourself apart from others, be open to opportunities, or make your own.

If you would like information on specialty leasing, you can write "Temporary Tenant" at P.O. Box 130, Jefferson Valley, NY 10535, or call them at (914) 739-3151, and they will send you three introductory issues of the newsletter for $9.

It's Your Choice...

The growth of your practice depends on what you want and where you want to go. You can have a laid-back, part-time practice where you work with just a few regular clients and collect a safe paycheck from another job. Or you can be so busy that you wish you had another pair of hands and a few more hours in the day.

Though the monetary compensation can be substantial, and the inner glow you get from knowing you have helped someone just seems to overflow the confines of your body, it isn't always a bed of roses. There will be times when your hands hurt so much that you can't even hold a pencil, your forearms feel weak, your neck and shoulder muscles go into spasm and you need a massage yourself. There will be times when you have a full day scheduled and then one by one your clients call to say something else came up, or worse yet, they don't call at all. There will be days when you don't have a full schedule, and horror of horrors, days when you don't have *any* clients. These are the valleys every self employed person has to face, but there are ways to level off these ups and downs.

While you are building your personal client base, supplement your income by working for someone else. Remember the health clubs, tanning studios, chiropractors' offices, swim clubs, cruise ships, wholistic centers. You can work with doctors on a referral basis, you can enter the sports field specializing in sports injuries, you can become a member of a traveling sportsmassage team and travel to such places as Dallas Texas, Washington, D.C. and Puerto Rico, all expenses paid. And the *crème de la crème* — you may be lucky enough to be part of the pro golf tours, or part of the entourage which accompanies entertainment stars on their tours, or wealthy people on their travels.

Establishing your reputation takes time. Your ethics, morals and rules of conduct must be above reproach. Your reputation precedes you. It can be the sweet smell of a rose garden or the stench of a garbage dump. Truly, you hold the success of your career in your hands.

PART TWO

Business Practices

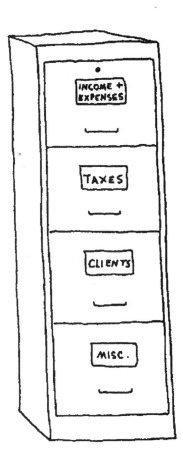

Being fun to do business with usually results in doing a lot more business.

--Author unknown

What Should I Charge?

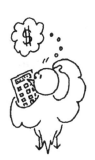

The bottom line — the big question. I have found that there is no hard and fast rule. The pay scale is varied and you can almost charge what the traffic will bear keeping in mind your experience, your expenses, your clientele, your stamina.

You will need enough start-up capital (money to buy your chair, a serviceable car, a suitable wardrobe). You need a good cash flow (money to pay expenses). You need operating money to meet your everyday expenses.

Just out of massage school I charged $35 an hour and thought I would never have the guts to charge $50 like my instructor did. Now I charge $55 an hour and $35 a half hour. This is within range for New York but might not hold true for other parts of the country.

If you are in doubt as to what to charge, call up other therapists in your area and inquire about their fees. You don't want to be *too* high or *too* low. Tell them you are a new therapist and don't want to undercut what they are charging. If anyone is asking a higher-than-the-norm fee, make an appointment for a massage (we can never get enough ourselves) and see what that therapist does that is different and warrants the higher fee. We can always learn from one another.

Now begin by taking an average of the fees. Then figure how many clients you need to see each week in order to meet your regular business and living expenses, based on that average. That's your bare minimum *survival level* of income — but it leaves nothing for emergencies, slow periods, or reinvestment in your practice. So add half again (at least) as many clients to your total, and *that* is how many clients you'd need to see in order to survive in your practice, at that fee scale.

If this number seems reasonable, great. You've just established your price. If it seems like an unreasonable number of clients to see each week, you'll need to charge more to make enough money to live. Or find a way to lower your cost of living, until you earn a reputation that will command the higher fee. The better your reputation, the more you will command, but you want your fee to be high enough to afford to give occasional discounts and investment-oriented freebies, or special price concessions for appropriate circumstances.

I work on a sliding scale, for example, for seniors and single working mothers. If a regular once-a-week client books two appointments in one week, I will give a 10% discount.

If I'm trying to draw back clients whom I haven't heard from in six months, I send a card offering a discount if they book by a certain date, generally three weeks down the line.

I offer my clients a 10% discount for any referrals they send me. When a person comes to me as a result of this referral, I make a note of that on my client's card so that I remember to honor the discount on their next visit.

If a client books four appointments in one month, they get a discount also. But the discount is not given until all four appointments have been kept.

Occasionally I have used the barter system to good advantage. I mentioned an impending move to a new apartment to one of my clients, and he told me in no uncertain terms that I was not to hire movers — he and his sons would take care of it. I, in turn, paid them with a massage.

A week later I was working on a new client who happened to be a carpet layer. He saw the rolled up carpet which I intended to lay in the office. How was I going to do it, I had no idea. He offered to lay it, stretch it and bind it for the price of a massage!

On Charging for On-Site Massage

For corporate, on-site massage, my regular fee is $25 for 15 minutes, for two or more people. The program can be paid for by the employer or by the employees.

If the employer is paying for the program, I write up a contract based on the number of people and the frequency of the massages. For a contract paid in full at the time of signing (always try to get your money up front), I will give a 10% discount. Otherwise payment is expected in 30 days.

If the employees are paying for their own massages, I will charge them $20 for 15 minutes, but a minimum of four is required to receive this discount. Remember, it does not pay you to travel any distance for just 15 minutes. Once again, get your money up front. Things do happen and people forget. If money has already been paid, there is less chance that the appointment won't be honored.

Of course, chair massage doesn't have to be limited to the corporate environment. If you choose to set up shop at a mall, flea market, craft show or the beach, the fee can be advertised at $1 a minute with the customer deciding the length of time. Set a kitchen timer in motion to keep track of the duration of the massage. If you do a good job, don't be surprised if your client asks for more time!

When I make a presentation to a company for on-site massage, I ask the decision maker to fill in the **Wellness In Business** form. You will then have a wealth of information at your fingertips:

QUESTION 1 is obvious.
QUESTION 2 tells you who your competitors are.
QUESTION 3 tells you what to delete or include in *your* program suggestions.
QUESTION 4 tells you how many days and how many therapists will be needed to provide your service.

WELLNESS IN BUSINESS SURVEY

1. Does your company offer a health promotion program to employees?
   ☐ Yes   ☐ No

2. If yes, who are the providers?
   ☐ In-house Staff   ☐ Community Center   ☐ Consultant
   ☐ Hospital   ☐ Fitness Center   ☐ Other

3. If yes, does the program contain any of the following components?
   ☐ Weight Control   ☐ Stress Management   ☐ Fitness
   ☐ Mini-Massage   ☐ Substance Abuse   ☐ Health Talks
   ☐ Nutritional Awareness

4. How many employees do your have? _____

5. What data do you collect that might be useful in evaluating employees' fitness/wellness?
   ☐ Absenteeism   ☐ Productivity
   ☐ Health Claims   ☐ Employee Turnover

6. What are the two most important reasons for your company to begin or continue a Health/Wellness program?
   ☐ Employee Morale   ☐ Cost Control
   ☐ Response to Employer Request   ☐ Corporate Image

7. With regard to cost control, which two of the following cost areas are most important to your company?
   ☐ Health Claims   ☐ Reduced Accidents
   ☐ Reduced Absenteeism   ☐ Improved Recruitment
   ☐ Improved Productivity   ☐ Improved Employee Retention

8. What do you consider the two most important barriers to initiating a Health/Wellness Promotion Program?
   ☐ Cost   ☐ Lack of Employee Commitment
   ☐ Liability   ☐ Lack of Expertise

9. Would you consider an employee interest survey as an important factor in your company's decision to initiate a Health/Wellness Promotion Program?
   ☐ Yes   ☐ No

61

Company Name: _____

EMPLOYEE SURVEY

Your company is considering implementing a Health/Wellness Promotion Program for its valued employees.

1. Would you support having:
   * a 15-minute "Mini-Massage" at your desk?   □ Yes □ No
   * half hour Health Enrichment Talks on:
      Nutrition . . . . □ Yes   □ No
      Stress--Good and Bad . . . . □ Yes   □ No
      Self Massage . . . . □ Yes   □ No
      Back Health . . . . □ Yes   □ No

2. What time of day would you most welcome a mini-break?
   □ Morning (10 to 12)   □ Noon (12 to 1)
   □ Afternoon (1 to 3)   □ End of day (3 to 5)
   □ Other _____

3. If your employer adopts this Wellness Program, would you be interested in attending voluntary Health Enrichment Talks, for a nominal fee per lecture, on subjects of your choice?
                    □ Yes   □ No
            Please check areas of interest:
   □ Nutritional Awareness   □ Reflexology
   □ Computer Fitness   □ Back to Basics
   □ Substance Abuse   □ Headaches
   □ Touch & Massage   □ Overuse Syndrome
   □ Hug Therapy   □ Your Healthy Heart
   □ Walk or Run?   □ Alone but Not Lonely
   □ Cry/Groan/Laugh -- Nature's Safety Valves
   □ Other _____

4. Would you like talks scheduled for:
   □ Once a Month   □ Twice a Month

5. If your company has Employee of the Month incentives, would you like to receive a free professional Swedish Massage?
   □ Yes   □ No

            Please return this survey to your Personnel Manager.

QUESTION 5 gives you an idea of where the employer is losing money and how your service can reverse the trend.

QUESTION 6 gives you an idea of his "hot" button — push it!

QUESTION 7 tells where he feels he can save money.

QUESTION 8 gives you his objections so you can overcome them.

QUESTION 9 will open the door for you to present the **Employee Survey** form.

The **Employee Survey** form will enable you to customize your program to meet the needs of the employees as well as prove to the employer that it would be a valued program to implement at his company. The Mini-Fix and Chair Massage flyers can be put up on the office bulletin board or in a lounge, if the employer doesn't want to pay for the program. Ask permission to do so.

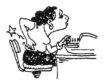

Get Yourself a MINI-FIX!

Do you ENJOY having bands of steel for shoulders?

Are you HAPPY with a bucket of hot coals in your low back?

Is an anvil chorus in your head your idea of soothing music?

We at TEN + TEN can help... Our licensed, energetic professionals will come to your office & administer a 15 minute, fully clothed chair massage to those areas which cause such distress during your workday.

You can give yourself ONE MINI FIX for $20, which can be applied towards package discounts. Keep a smile on your face!

SHORT CIRCUIT STRESS BEFORE IT BECOMES DIS-STRESS...

Chair Massage

Do you have tension?
Do you have stress?
Let me show you
What is best...

The best is massage
Done on a chair.
No oil - fully clothed -
Can be done anywhere.

Mental sharpness is enhanced,
Concentration doubles.
One little mini-massage
Will soothe away your troubles.

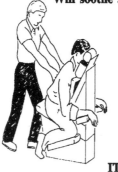

15 Minutes
$20

Your Business Card

IT'S GREAT TO BE KNEADED

Flyers can be posted on bulletin boards in employee lounges to advertise your on-site massage service. But get the employer's permission first.

Using Incentives

I have taken a tip from my local photo shop — the owner gives a card to his customers, which is punched each time the customer does business with him. After a certain number of punches, you get a free roll of film, reprints at half price, or 10% off the price of developing (I'm not the only 10%er around!). You can be sure I patronize that shop rather than the one that is nearer to me but where I don't get such premiums.

So I devised a card for each of my clients, which I keep a copy of with their records. As they come for their

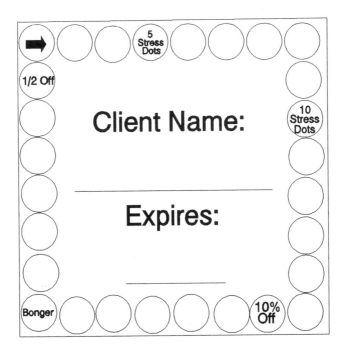

treatment, I punch both cards, the one for my office files and the one I give them so they can keep track of their progress. I use two cards to prevent fraudulent punches and to keep track in case they lose or forget theirs.

The card has a total of 28 circles to punch out. In the fourth circle, I give five Stressdots. In the tenth circle, I give a strip of 10 Stressdots. In the 16th circle, I give 10% off an hour massage. In the 22nd circle, I give a Bonger. In the 28th circle, I give 50% off an hour massage. This incentive card promotes loyalty and gets them in the habit of coming on a regular basis.

I don't feel I am being unprofessional because I sometimes adjust my fees, or offer discounts or free give-aways. We are in a giving, caring profession and this is my way of showing my clients that I have their interests at heart, especially in difficult economic times. It's part of being true to basic human values, and being an ethical human being.

Tips and Ethics

Of course, there is always a welcome plus in the form of a tip. I know many therapists abhor the idea of accepting a tip as being unprofessional. After all, doctors and dentists don't accept tips. Though I consider myself a professional, I am also in the service business, and as such I feel complimented when a client wishes to express his pleasure by offering me something extra. I know some therapists who go so far as to put "no tips" on their business cards. Everyone has to decide what they are most comfortable with and take it from there. Needless to say, a tip is *never* accepted for sexual favors!

A goal for all therapists should be ethical relationships between client and therapist, as well as between therapist and therapist. Whatever you decide to charge, make it fair to yourself, to your clients, and to other practicing therapists. Being cutthroat has no place in our healing profession. And word does get around.

Become friends with your fellow therapists. You'll find the support very comforting when you feel you have been cut adrift in the turbulent sea of free enterprise.

One other thing I do when a colleague comes to me for massage is to give a "professional discount." (There I go with my 10% discount again!). Believe me, whatever I give out returns to me two-fold if not in money, then in good-will and friendship. I feel good about myself, my clients are happy, and my business prospers.

Choose a job you love, and
you will never have to work
a day in your life.

--Confucius

Keeping Records

The second worst phrase in the English language after "death and taxes" has got to be "keeping records." Much as we hate to do it, it is necessary to placate Uncle Sam and to keep us on track with our business. It's what is known as "being organized." Once you find a system that you are happy with, you'll find that the required paperwork will actually make your work easier.

You will need a system for keeping financial records, a system for making and tracking appointments, and a system to organize client information. In addition, you may need to file for certain business licenses, and you'll need to keep insurance coverage to protect yourself and your business.

Keeping It Legal and Safe

Legally establishing a business usually involves more than hanging out a sign. Before declaring yourself open for business, check the local and state requirements. Papers may need to be filed with the state, along with a small fee. Local zoning restrictions may determine whether you can operate out of home, or if you need a zoned business location.

The U.S. Small Business Administration is a good first stepping stone to familiarize yourself with such requirements. They publish several informative pamphlets (such as a *Checklist for Going into Business*), and often hold local meetings to help new business owners get started.

By calling 1-800-827-5722 in Washington, D.C., you will reach the SBA's Small Business Answer Desk. From a touch-tone phone you can access any of several pre-recorded messages on topics such as Starting Your Own Business, SBA Services and Local Assistance, Woman's Business Ownership, and others. You will also be able to obtain the phone number of your local SBA office by listening to the message on SBA Services and Local Assistance, and following their directions. A prerecorded message will give you the local SBA office based on the area code you enter. From there you can receive a startup kit and personal assistance.

The 800- number is a quick and handy way to obtain a great deal of information, but for those who prefer to let their feet do the walking a trip to the public library is the answer. The reference librarian can direct you to the vertical files, which should contain all or most of the SBA's 50-plus publications.

To obtain information on your local ordinances, you may contact your city hall, county courthouse or state Small Business office.

When I started up I relied on books such as *The Woman's Guide to Starting a Business* by Claudia Jessup and Genie Chipps, which can be a helpful resource and a good addition to your personal library. Other materials I found helpful are listed in the APPENDIX.

Most new business guides advise obtaining an attorney, who may prove to be a valuable counselor for reviewing contract agreements, leases, release forms you may want to use, etc. As you begin making money and keeping financial records, a good accountant can steer you through the maze of tax laws and forms. (Someone once said, "It's not how much you make, but how much you *keep* that counts." Probably an accountant.)

Finally, it is always wise to protect your investment with proper insurance. Being self employed full time means you will need to provide your own benefits package — health insurance, life insurance, disability coverage — in addition to liability insurance. Check your homeowners or renters insurance policy to see if it will cover your important equipment and supplies for fire, theft, etc.

Team Work

It is extremely important to keep good records, especially if there is a team working corporate massage. Credibility, responsibility and dependability are of the utmost importance in building an on-site business. You need a "hunter" to find prospects, you need a "bird dog" to flush the sales and you need a "retriever" to bring back the contracts. You need a director to train the team and send them on the assignments. You need a manager to make sure the team is making their assigned rounds. You need a bookkeeper to keep track of monies coming in from contracts and monies paid to the team members.

This type of enterprise has to be run the same way any other business is run. If you are a sole proprietor, *you* wear all the hats. If you have a partnership, the work can be divided up, each partner working where he is most comfortable. In an "S" Corporation, all tasks can be shared with *compatible* members. In a one person operation, you do all the work but the profits belong to you alone. In a group endeavor, the work is divided but so are the profits.

Keeping Client Records

After much experimenting and revising, I settled on a system which worked well for me, and yet is a simple and inexpensive way to start. I have included samples of this beginning system and hope it will serve as a starting point for you. Client record-keeping systems can get very elaborate and expensive, but for a small or a beginning practice it is a needless waste of money and time — wait to invest in a more elaborate system until the size of your practice warrants the investment.

The very least information you need concerning your client is, of course, his/her name, address, telephone number and how your name was obtained — referral, yellow pages (if you advertise there), gift certificate, etc. Why is this information important? If it's a referral, you will want to thank the person making the referral (common courtesy). If from the yellow pages or any other type of advertising, you will want to know where your advertising dollars are being used most effectively, thereby saving you money. If you find Gift Certificates or other discount promotions are profitable, then you will want to capitalize on that information by sending out flyers periodically.

To keep your system in order, get the largest ring binder you can find, a supply of alphabetized index dividers, and a supply of manila pocket sheets to hold your Client Information Card, Treatment Record Sheet, and Health Questionnaire.

Client Information Card.

On the Client Information Card I have a line for Date of Birth (I send birthday cards), Height and Weight (so I know how much energy I will require to complete the treatment — I have found that in order not to burn out I have to pace myself very carefully), a disclaimer so the client knows I am not going beyond the limits of my training, a line for them to sign their name so I know they have read it and the date to document their first visit.

In order to prevent paper clutter, I transfer the information they have given me on the Health Questionnaire to the back of the Client Information Card. Then I can throw the questionnaire away. At the bottom of the card, on the back, I write down the fee I charged, whether it was discounted in some way, and the year that fee was charged (in case you raise the price). I also record any tip I may have received.

On your client card, highlight specific preferences of your clients. Does she want a pillow under her head? Does he prefer cream over oil? Does he feel seasick when you play your sailboat tape? Does she want a cloth over her eyes? Are his feet ticklish?

Did she just have a new grandchild? Make note of the birth date and the name. You will endear yourself forever to this proud grandparent when you make inquiries into the progress of little Rebecca or Robert.

Is his darling daughter getting married? Make a note on your calendar and send a congratulatory card *to Mom and Dad*.

If a client requests that you send no correspondence or call them at home, mark the card in RED so you will remember to comply with his wishes. Ask if it will be okay to contact him at his place of business, and if he says yes, use discretion when the receptionist asks the purpose of your call.

HEALTH QUESTIONNAIRE
In order that we may better serve you, please answer the following:

Do you have arthritis? Where:_____

Do you have headaches or sinus trouble? _____

Do you have heart related ailments? _____

Do you have diabetes/hypoglycemia? _____

Do you suffer with backache? Where:_____

Have you had any broken bones/fractures? Where:_____

Have you had neck/shoulder pain? _____

Are you fatigued/nervous/depressed? _____

Do you smoke? _____ Is your circulation poor? _____

Do you have high/low blood pressure? _____

Is gas/constipation/diarrhea a problem? _____

Do you have allergies? What kind:_____

Do you have varicose veins/phlebitis? _____

Have you had any operations? For what:_____

Is your range of motion limited in any way? _____

Do you wear contacts/dentures? _____

Are you pregnant? (Women only!) _____

Do you exercise regularly? _____ Favorite sport (if any):_____

Have you been massaged before? _____

What is your occupation? _____
                              THANK YOU

Date   **TREATMENT ATTENDANCE RECORD**

MUSIC

Showing you care makes your clients feel that they are very special to you and so they should be, whether they are the client whose fee has remained the same as when you first went into business or the client who tips generously each time he comes for a treatment. I have both kinds and one balances off the other.

On the Treatment Attendance Record, I write in the date I saw them, where I found spasms and tension, where they told me they hurt, what I did and the title of the cassette that I played during the treatment. I play a different tape each session, and by the time we go through the whole repertoire they have picked out their favorites. Knowing that allows me to provide yet another service for them. One client loves the ocean so whenever he is scheduled for a visit, "his" tape is in the cassette, ready to go. I also jot down any interesting facts we may have spoken about and refer back to them on the next visit. This demonstrates to the client that you care about them and what's going on in their lives.

To further define your client record and to flag the birthday month for sending birthday cards, put an index tab on the top of the manila pocket sheet that contains your client's Information Card and Treatment Attendance Record. Mark the tab with a large J for January, F for February, etc., through the year.

About two weeks before January birthdays, go through your looseleaf book and write out all those cards. On the front of the pocket, make a note of what card you sent and the date it was sent. If you are using original cards, as I do, this prevents your sending the same card each year. I do the same when sending Christmas cards.

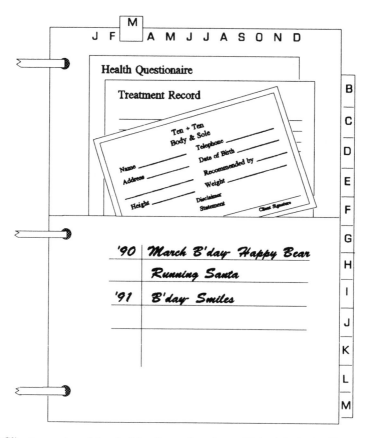

Client records notebook. Manila pocket sheets filed alphabetically (tabs on right) hold client information. Tabs on top indicate month of birth. Cards sent are noted on the pocket front.

In the corner where the stamp will go, I write the date that the card is to be mailed — usually three days before the actual birthday (example: 1-3-92 for a January 5th birthday). Then all my January rememberences are rubber-banded together and mailed out on the appropriate day. (I keep track of paying my bills this way also.)

Because my clientele has outgrown the confines of the looseleaf book method, I am now using the Safeguard Business System (order a free brochure by writing Safeguard Business Systems, Inc., 455 Maryland Drive, Fort Washington, PA., 19034). I redesigned the original system to fit the needs of a massage practice. It follows the basic format described for the looseleaf method, but is more extensive and allows for more flexibility.

I approached this system cautiously and took it in small steps because it is expensive to set up. But I am extremely pleased with its organizational capabilities and the sense of order it has brought to my business. If you plan on staying in the massage profession, I heartily recommend it — it is well worth the money.

My first small step was to buy their Economy Rack. I was able to test my system, and once I realized it would work I ordered my first modular unit with its stand. It is a beautiful piece of furniture and does much to add to the professional appearance of my office. The Economy Rack is still used — by my secretary when she needs to take a large number of files out to work on.

In the Safeguard System, the file pouch (essentially a specially die-cut file folder, with closed ends to prevent papers from falling out) holds the Client Information Cards and Treatment Attendance Records. A clear plastic holder slips over the top of the file pouch, allowing it to hang in the file drawer, like a standard hanging file folder.

On the plastic top holder, I place a pink name label for women and a blue name label for men. My clients are place alphabetically according to a color code, with red tabs indicating names beginning with A, yellow tabs signifying the letter B, blue tabs for the letter C, and so on through the alphabet. Notches on the top of the plastic file holder assure you of lining up the tabs properly. At the far left side of the plastic holder I put the year label. Since each year comes in a different color, I can keep track of when my clients first came to me.

In the Information Section (Section 2 in the illustration), which has four notches in which I can place identifying tabs, I use yellow tabs to denote clients who have come to me through the yellow pages. Clients that I have gotten as a result of advertising other than yellow pages are so noted with purple tabs. The next slots to the right are for those clients who have come because of referrals — those tabs are green. Next, I use blue tabs to indicate clients that have come to me through spas, fitness centers, salons, tanning and toning places. Finally, black tabs indicate clients from hotels.

In the Follow-Up Section (Section 3), I make note of the birth month with brown tabs. At the far right of the plastic heading I use a colored marker tab to flag clients who owe me money or Insurance payments that are outstanding. I'm sure you can appreciate the wealth of information this system puts at your fingertips — visually, without ever having to remove a file from it place in your rack.

You can think of the Safeguard System as providing

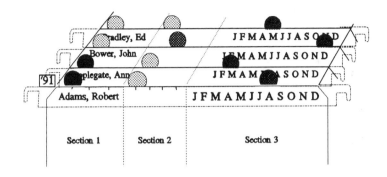

The Safeguard System with color-coded tabs. Section 1 is the Identification Section. Different colored tabs indicate where the A's end and the B's begin. Section 2 is the Information Section. Here a yellow tab indicates the client came through the yellow pages, while green-tabbed client was a referral, and a purple-tabbed client came from any other source of advertising, etc. This is an excellent way to track the effectiveness of your advertising and promotional dollars. Section 3 is the Follow-Up Section. As a dedicated sender of greeting cards, I find this section invaluable for flagging birthdays.

you with a "visual database" of information, by the appropriate placement of colored tabs along the top edge of each client's file pouch.

Your Appointment System

After each treatment, I ask WHEN (positive thinking!) they want to schedule their next appointment and I enter it in the large desk appointment book. Having a large desktop appointment book that shows the times in hourly increments makes it easy for me to work with. If an appointment is on the half or the quarter hour, I just write it in for that time.

81

Try to schedule new people on the half hour, and book your regulars on the hour. Over-book. Get the phone number of the new client and then call back to confirm the number — and always write the appointment in pencil until it is confirmed. This will save considerable aggravation for you if they don't show. There are those undesirables who deny their interest is in manual release, and will book the appointment, then get back at you by not showing up. You will also be able to ascertain whether the number is legitimate, or just the figment of their fertile imaginations. Give your established clientele preference over new people. For a more detailed description and explanation of scheduling times for new or questionable clients, see the section on "The Chronic Late-Comer/No Show" on page 155.

Instead of carrying around the Big Book, I use a calendar sheet from a desk blotter, folded to fit in my pocketbook. It is large, has lots of lines to write time and name of client, plus my own social dates. Clients are written in green and personal engagements in red — a quick and easy method to keep track of your life. And your calendar always looks full!

Just remember to transfer any appointments you make while you are out of the office into your desk appointment book, and vice-versa.

I have had Appointment Reminder cards made up, on which I put the date and time of clients' next appointments, with the request that they call should they be unable to keep their date. Make sure you have your name and telephone number on the pad.

Some therapists have an appointment reminder printed on the back of their business cards — a very good idea also.

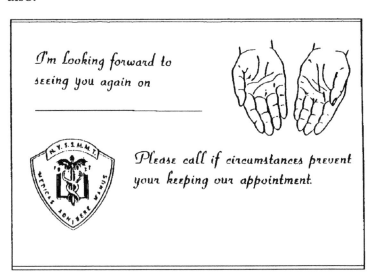

I'm looking forward to seeing you again on

_____

Please call if circumstances prevent your keeping our appointment.

Financial Record Keeping

I have chosen not to accept reimbursement through insurance companies in my practice, for three reasons: first, not all insurance companies cover massage therapy; second, companies can take a long time to pay and be a pain to deal with; and third, it greatly simplifies my record keeping by dealing directly with the paying client only.

Some therapists do a big business through medical insurance reimbursement. More power to them. I choose not to get involved in the headaches of it all, but if you want to go that route for your practice, a good resource for you would be the *Insurance Reimbursement Manual* (see the APENDIX for the address and phone number to order).

I ask my clients to pay me as services are rendered, and ask them to seek reimbursement directly from their own insurance company if they would like to. If any of my clients want a receipt for insurance purposes, I use the form printed with the name of my company and address, and after the words "Neuromuscular Therapy," I add, "as prescribed by Dr. _____."
I give my clients a copy of the "Statement of Medical Necessity" letter, and tell them to have their doctor or

---

Statement of Medical Necessity Form
Doctor's Letterhead

Date

___(Patient's Name)___ has been referred for conservative treatment of his/her ____(Disease/Condition)____ to __(Your Name & License #)__ for Neuromuscular Therapy. He/she has suffered with ___(Problem)___ as a result of his/her ____(Doctor's diagnosis)____ , and should respond favorably to this treatment, in conjunction with standard medical procedures.

Sincerely,

Dr._____

Insurance Code #97145, Neuromuscular Therapy

---

chiropractor type it on the doctor's letterhead, filling in the pertinent information. This, along with my receipt for services rendered, is mailed to the client's insurance carrier for reimbursement.

As I said, this greatly reduces my time and expense in terms of record keeping, billing and tracking.

To keep track of my weekly *expenses and receipts*, I use **Dome's Simplified Weekly Bookkeeping Record**, which is widely available in almost any office supply store, and even in most well-supplied drug stores. I find the breakdown of expenditures very concise. Not all of their categories apply to our profession, but those that do make it easy on me when my accountant questions where the money went.

The *Dome* book includes a brief section of "Special Instructions for Professional Men and Women" which itemizes many of the allowable deductions we can take. Some of the listed deductions include cost of supplies, rent paid for office rooms, cost of fuel, water, light, and telephone used in offices, cost of furniture, books, automobile usage, etc. It certainly pays to keep a good record of these things — I.R.S. requires *everything* to be documented properly, but these necessary professional expenses are legitimate deductions and certainly should be figured carefully. No sense paying more in taxes than Uncle Sam requires. Consult a good accountant for specific help in your situation.

I supplement the Dome system (for tracking expenses) with a Daily Income Log (for tracking income). I have adapted mine from a "Daily Business Income Log" form designed by Jefferson Saunders, L.M.P. (It is one of several forms he has designed and assembled in a *Record*

Year 1991   Month August   # Clients Seen _____   Gross Income _____   Page __ / of __

Date	Client Name	Fee	Cash	Check	Charge	Hotel	Lecture	Work-shops	Gift Cert.	Dis-count	Tips
1st	D. Leo	100.-	✓								
	E. Shifflet	35.-	✓								
	WEEKLY TOTAL	(135.-)									
5th	S. Smith	60.-	✓								
	J. Hedges	40.-	✓								
	R. Rogers	-							✓		
	L. Dunbar	105.-	✓						✓		
6th	R. Ruff	60.-	✓								
	L. Concetta	65.-		✓							
	G. Davids	55.-	✓								
7th	C. Thomas	35.-	✓								
	WEEKLY TOTAL	(420)									

Daily Income Log. Subtotal by week, then calculate the overall total for each month.

Keeping for Massage Professionals package which he sells for $18, available from N.E.I. Publishing and Marketing, PO Box 20445, Seattle, WA., 98102). This log is an in depth breakdown of clients and receipts, tallied by week and by month. This record tells me who I saw, the date I saw them, the fee charged, how it was paid, and where I conducted the business (hotel, workshops, giving a talk or lecture, etc.). I also document whether it was a Gift Certificate, if a discount was given, and also my tips.

I transfer my monthly totals to a standard ledger to document the year by month for several years. (For you who are very competitive, you can order a "Beat Yesterday" ledger from Sales Record Publishing Company, Inc., P.O. Box 206, Pomfret, CT., 06258, which breaks down income trends year to year *by the week* and the month.) By keeping these year-to-year records, you can see if you are ahead of what you did last year, holding your own, or (horrors!) falling behind. It will also show you when your ups and downs occur during the year. The ledger would look like this:

	1989	1990	1991
January	3,099.50	2,713.50	2,950.00
February	2,876.00	2,692.85	2,707.40
March	2,998.00	3,142.45	3,015.25
December	2,617.81	3,158.00	3,010.25
TOTAL FOR YEAR	32,138.50	35,037.80	36,819.45

If you find July is consistently slow, you can either take a vacation yourself, or you can change your physical location and follow your fellow sun worshippers, and head for the resorts. Of course, make these arrangements far in advance of the season in order to secure a spot for yourself.

If you fancy yourself a true child of nature, head for the beaches with your table and "rub" away! Just be sure sand is not a part of your oil concoction — you want to soothe tender skin, not peel it like an onion.

One of my clients related the "sad" tale of the therapist he met in Maui, Hawaii. She held court under the palm trees at the beach and did her thing until the surfing waves departed the area at the end of the season. She then packed her gear and headed for the ski resorts in France for the winter. Have hands, will travel! What a way to go.

While you are doing all this traveling, be it domestic or foreign, don't forget to keep a travel log of your expenses. If you use a car, get an Auto Milage Record Book and be faithful in recording distances traveled, areas covered, oil and gas expenditures, plus repair and maintenance costs. All these facts are deductible on your income tax, but they must be substantiated.

The final record I keep is a Gift Certificate Register. You not only can track revenue from Gift Certificates, but it also allows you to check off certificates which have been sold and redeemed. You will be amazed at how your income can increase through this avenue alone.

GIFT CERTIFICATE REGISTER							
Date Sold	Exp. Date	Presented by	Issued to	Amt.	1/2 hr.	Hr.	Date Re-dmd

I imagine by now you are throwing up your hands, ready to chuck the whole business. But take heart. You can't eat an elephant in one bite (even if you had a taste for elephant), but you could, one bite at a time! Go slowly, take it a little at a time. You may not be inclined to use all the records which I have described, you may be inspired to develop different types of records (especially if you are computer-minded). Or you may choose not to keep records at all — not a very good idea, but you are your own boss and as such you can direct your own destiny. Good luck!

It takes less effort to keep
an old client satisfied than
to get a new client interested.

--Polish proverb

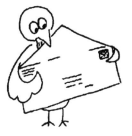

Keeping "In Touch"

The first secret to establishing excellent client relationships is to give the very best treatment you can, every time your hands contact their bodies. Keep in mind actors on the stage — the day *you* view the show may be the 100th time *they* have performed the part, but it is the first time *you* have seen it.

Your personal problems, *your* health concerns, *your* lack of energy have no place at your treatment table. You have to be there for your client. If you aren't, he will sense it and you will be giving less than your best.

It has happened to me. My client offered to give ME a shoulder rub! Another time I was bursting with energy — my client felt it and gave me a tip over and above the usual amount, saying he knew I had given him something special and he wanted to show me how much he appreciated it.

Secret number two: Simple consideration and caring. How seldom we really *communicate* with each other. Does your client feel that you see a dollar sign when you look at him? And they you have no more thought of him once he closes your office door? I know how much I love to be remembered on my birthday, and I want to do something to pass along that feeling to my clients.

I wanted them to know how special they are to me, so I began designing original greeting cards with a massage theme. All of a sudden, a satellite business was born.

It turned out to be a "double whammy" — clients call to say my card was the ONLY card they had received (talk about making points!), and then they would tell me they had been thinking of calling for an appointment but kept forgetting (don't we *all* have busy schedules?). And so, with card still in hand, they call to say "Thank you," and then book an appointment before they forget again.

The cards I send are not glossy, many-colored master-pieces, but the originality of the thought is what my clients appreciate. How often have *you* called someone to thank them for your birthday remembrance? A card that stands out, for whatever reason, gets comments.

This appreciative response stimulated me to expand on the idea. I have added Holiday greetings, discounts for booking within a certain time (generally during my slow periods), a card "just for no reason" (aren't these the best kind?), Gift Certificates (these have increased business during the holiday season). I have cards that remind them that I have not seen them for a while (what's new? are they okay?), and I have a card that just says, "I miss U."

Below are some samples of cards that I have used — make up your own, or you can order an assorted set of 12 (including those below) from the sheet on the last page of the book.

Everybody likes to know they are cared about. Yes, thoughtfulness DOES PAY OFF!

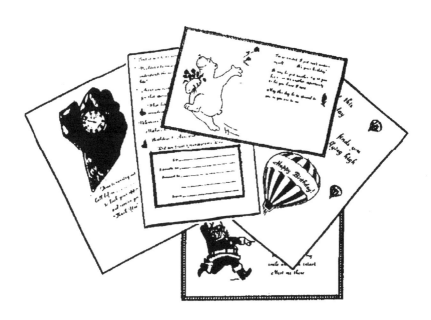

PART THREE

Professional Ethics

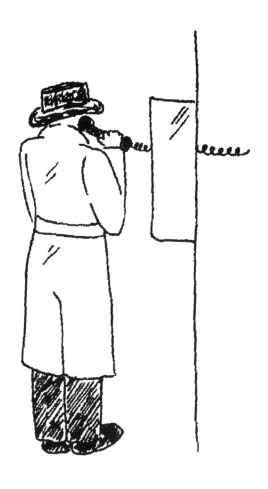

Crack up with laughter
before you crack up with
stress.

--Unknown

Handling Questionable Calls

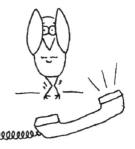

One of the most distressing aspects of our profession is the screening and handling of prospective clients. This has proven so stressful to some female therapists that in order not to have to deal with the situation, they limit their practice to women only, men on referral. Next to burnout and Carpal Tunnel Syndrome, this problem causes many therapists to give up their work.

So what can we do about it — is there a solution other than changing professions?

To answer that question, I would like to give you two telephone scripts that I've developed. The longer version may cause you discomfort — "I could never say that" will probably be your first reaction. But believe me, as harsh or "unlady-like" as it may sound, I have found that I could not beat around the bush with my replies, I had to let them know that I knew what they wanted and I had to let them know in no uncertain terms, that my practice was legal and ethical.

During busy seasons I have hired teenagers to help out in the office. Rather than subject them to any uncomfortable encounters with the seedy side of humanity, I give them the following script to follow:

ANSWERING THE TELEPHONE
- SHORT VERSION -

Receptionist: (name of your company), *Kim speaking.*

Caller: *I'd like to make an appointment.*

Receptionist: *Have you been here before?*

If the answer is NO — say: *The therapist is busy just now, but if you'll give me your name and telephone number, I'll have her call you as soon as she's free.*

If the answer is YES — Take their name and telephone number and ask if they would like an hour or a half hour appointment, and what day and time they would like to come in. Then enter the information in the desk appointment book.

IF THEY WANT ANY INFORMATION CONCERNING MY SERVICES OR WHAT KIND OF MASSAGE I DO, say: *THE THERAPIST WILL CALL YOU BACK TO GIVE YOU THAT INFORMATION.* (Don't forget to ask for the name and number).

Caller: *What does it cost?*

Receptionist: *$55 an hour or $35 a half hour — by appointment.*

If they want to know ANYTHING ELSE, say: *You will have to speak to the therapist.*

Caller: *Where are you located?*

Receptionist: (give name of street and town).

If they want more detail, say: *The therapist will give you further directions when you make your appointment.*

Receptionist: *Thank you for calling.*

ANSWERING THE TELEPHONE
- LONGER VERSION -

Therapist: (name of your company), *Maryann speaking.*

Caller: *I'd like some information about massage.*

Therapist: *We do Medical (I like to start with that as it helps establish the tone), Sports, Reflexology and Therapeutic Swedish.*

Caller: *What's the difference?*

Therapist: *Medical is generally one half hour and is done through a referral from a Doctor or Chiropractor. Sports, again, is generally a half hour and is done to prevent or cure sports injuries. Reflexology is a half hour treatment on the reflexes on the feet. These reflexes relate to all the organs and parts of the body. Therapeutic Swedish Massage uses five different techniques to knead and relax the muscles. For the relief of stress and tension, it's best to book an hour.*

Caller: *What's it cost?*

Therapist: *$55 an hour and $35 a half hour.*

Caller: *Is it a FULL body massage?*

Therapist: *Yes, with the exception of the genitals.*

Caller: *Do you accept tips?* (Meaning: for manual release).

Therapist: *No, we do not.*

Caller: *What do I wear? Do I have to be covered?*

Therapist: *You remove your clothing but are completely covered with a sheet towel.*

Caller: *But I don't like to be covered — I've had massage where I haven't been covered.*

Therapist: *In New York State it's the law that the genitals be covered. If you insist on being uncovered then I can't accept you as a client.*

Caller: *Even if I give you $100?*

Therapist: *Absolutely not — good-by!*

I have been asked if I massage topless, how old I am, what I look like, if I did "nude mutual." I answer: "What does any of that have to do with the quality of my massage?", and then I hang up.

Unfortunately, the massage parlor types are becoming more sophisticated with their questions and knowledgeable of the answers we will give them, so a few will slip by the initial telephone screening.

The next plateau they have to overcome is the Client Information Card and Health Questionnaire. If they refuse to fill them out then I tell them I can't take them as a client because the "law" requires that I keep records. I have had several people walk out at this point. I have had those who fill out the forms giving incorrect addresses and phone numbers. These are weeded out the first time I send them a Birthday Card or Christmas Card which is returned as "unknown." Another plus for "keeping in touch."

At the completion of one massage, a client asked, "Is that all?" When I said yes, he replied, "You're the only one I've ever gone to who didn't give release at the end." I told him I never said I did, and I don't! (Toss HIS card in the trash).

Another unpleasant encounter was with a nicely dressed gentleman. My secretary had booked him, giving him all the required information. Even so, he made suggestive remarks during the massage. At the end, because he didn't get what he was hinting for, he refused to give me the full fee, saying that what he offered was the fee quoted him by my secretary. I know what he

101

said was untrue, but rather than risk him walking out without paying at all, I accepted the money. Another lesson learned the hard way. Now I ask for payment after they fill out the forms and before they get on the table. Needless to say, his card was duly noted and put in the "dead file."

Joe Salerno, a retired dentist who now devotes himself to the wholistic way of life through massage/yoga therapy, says that as for those female clients "coming on" to him, he tells them he is very flattered but that he is a professional and such conduct could ruin his reputation and jeapordize his license.

Another reason for always conducting your business in an ethical manner is the possibility of a visit from an undercover agent...(nice play on words, don't you think?).

A well dressed man booked an appointment with me, looked at the diplomas I had on the wall and remarked on the number of "credentials" I had. A dead give away, as most people don't use that particular word. When I gave him the forms, he objected to the amount of "paperwork" he had to fill out. When I told him it was required by law, he made some excuse about not having the time for the massage and left.

Once again I had a visit from a gentleman who looked at the forms, filled them out and then said he had to make a phone call to the office. When I offered him the use of my phone, he said it was long distance and he preferred to call from outside. . .and besides, he was parked illegally and wanted to move his car. P.S....he never came back!

I have written about these two examples because at the time of their visits, the police were investigating and closing massage parlors throughout the area. There is something to be said about having a clear conscience. As long as you are conducting your business in an honest, professional manner, you have nothing to fear.

PART FOUR

Therapist
Heal Thyself

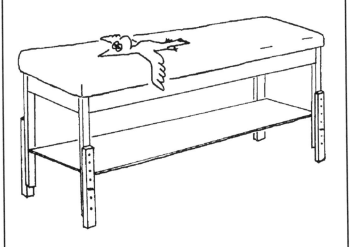

Think young. Aging is for wine.

--Unknown

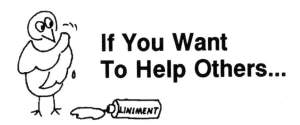

If You Want
To Help Others...

The most important person in the client/practitioner partnership is you. If you aren't in the best of health, how can you expect to help others?

We are in the business of helping those who seek out our expertise, but how many of us remember to take care of ourselves. Being on our feet all day can be exhausting... an exhausted therapist is an ineffectual therapist.

As a professional business person, you need to make sure to protect your most valuable asset — yourself!

Of course, everyone knows to bend at the knees and keep the back straight, don't you? If you've forgotten that cardinal rule, put a sign up in a prominent place as a reminder. If you don't, you'll find yourself looking for another career, or worse yet, the tables will be turned and *you* will be the recipient instead of the giver.

Chiropractors advise those who stand a lot to place one foot on a box or stool. This helps maintain the spine's

107

three curves and prevents fatigue. I use a small foot stool which I can move along by pushing it with one foot. It slips out of sight under the table when not in use.

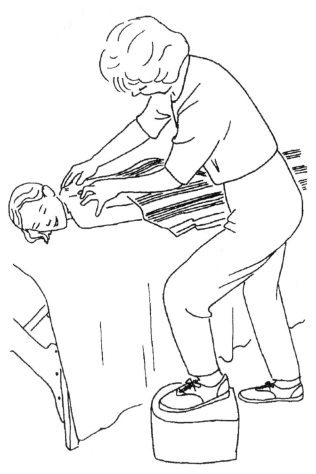

Place your foot on a box or a small stool while working to help prevent back fatigue.

It also helps my senior and/or infirm clients on and off the table more easily. If you know anyone handy enough to nail a piece of board on top of four legs (9 1/2 inches high), ask them to contribute their skill for the advancement of your career. Otherwise you can search the department stores for a suitable stool. If all else fails, order from the Darby Drug Company, 100 Banks Avenue, Rockville Centre, NY 11571 (phone number 800 247-4768), and ask for chrome frame stool, #700-8-990, 9 1/2 in. Cost: $24.95. Caution — don't use a stool with wheels, which could cause the stool to slip out from under the feet, especially if your office is not carpeted.

I keep a higher stool at the head of the table so I can sit while doing the neck, shoulders, and face. To conserve energy, sit whenever possible.

Burn out is a very real occupational hazard in our profession. The number one rule for survival is learning how to pace yourself. I ask my secretary to leave 15 or 30 minutes between appointments. This allows time for my client to rest a few minutes before getting dressed. It also gives me a breather so I can recoup my energy.

A worthwhile and, to me, necessary investment, is a high back recliner. It serves double duty as my desk chair. The fifteen to thirty minutes between appointments gives me time for quiet meditation and deep breathing. The high back affords me a place to rest my head and the reclining ability of the chair allows my body to fully relax within a short space of time.

For those of you just starting out who have to hustle and don't have the luxury of scheduling your own time,

I suggest taking at least five minutes to stretch, shake out your hands, bend over to get the blood back into your brain, and close your eyes. If you have been going at full stream all day, dip your hands into cold water to reduce any swelling. Five minutes lying on the floor in the yoga corpse position, is also helpful in overcoming fatigue.

By scheduling 15 to 30 minutes as a buffer between appointments, I am insuring against "client pile up." *I* hate waiting and therefore I give my clients the courtesy of taking *them* on time. Since I don't have a formal waiting room in my office, if I happen to be running late, I leave a note on the door of my office informing them of the delay. There is a chair for them to sit on if they have to wait. While I am working I set the hands of a time clock (attached to the door) to the time I will be free. I've also had a sign made which reads "In session, please wait." This lets any unexpected visitors know that I am in the office.

Time is an elusive commodity -- it tends to get away from us. Traffic can be unpredictable, emergencies can arise at the last moment, appointments can be over-looked. The 15 to 30 minute "window" allows for people who are always early (like myself) and for people who are chronically late. A good deal of stress for you can be avoided by not booking too tightly. If a late-comer's arrival intrudes on a following client's time, they know that their treatment time will be shortened so as not to penalize the client who is on time.

In order to prevent missed appointments, confirm the day before. I neglected to do this for a "regular" who didn't show up. She had gotten caught up with bill paying and had completely forgotten the time. Luckily I was able to reschedule her. She was so apologetic for the inconvenience she had caused me that she arrived with a beautiful rose and a note saying, "Thank you for being so nice." Here's an example of the therapist receiving some stroking. Could I have gotten angry and upset? Yes, I could have... but who would have suffered? As it turned out, we *both* were happy little campers.

On the other hand there are those who book, give you a name and telephone number and then don't show up. I have had whole days fall apart because of this lack of consideration. But I had no one to blame but myself. If I had called I would have discovered that the name was fictitious, the number was not in service or there was no such party at that telephone number. Do I blow up? I used to, especially when I saw unpaid bills where fees should have been. Lesson learned — don't put yourself in such a vulnerable position... *confirm!*

I wrote earlier about remembering to bend the knees and keep the back straight. Now I want to discuss keeping the wrists straight and the fingers flexible.

To give support to the wrist while doing effleurage, I wrap one hand around the working wrist. I am able to exert deeper pressure without straining or bending the wrist. Instead of

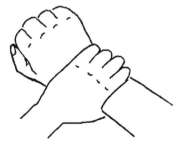

using the heel of your hand, which can lead to carpal tunnel syndrome, keep your wrist in a neutral position and use your knuckles. Here again, you will find you are able to use more pressure. I find this position most helpful when working on a client who has very tight skin.

I do effleurage on the back stroking from the head to the waist. At one time I positioned myself near the top of my client's head. I have many long-torsoed clients which caused me to stretch beyond my comfort zone, and I found myself suffering with backaches. Necessity is the mother of invention, so I moved my body from the central head position to the area of the client's shoulder. Presto — no more stretching and no more backaches.

While working the erector spinae along the length of the spine, I support my fingers by grasping the phalanges of the working hand with the fingers of my other hand. This acts as a splint and allows me to apply as much pressure as is needed. Quite a few of my clients are very tight in the mid thoracic area. After loosening the muscles along the spine with my finger technique, I concentrate additional pressure on the thoracic area with my thumb. Caution — make sure your nails are *short*.

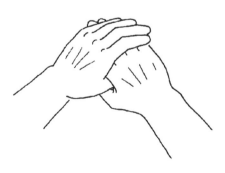

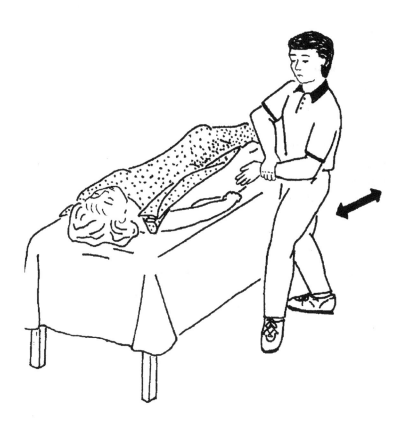

When working on the right tensor fascia lata, I place my left elbow in my left hip, hold my left wrist with my right hand and rock my whole body forward and backward as a unit. As I move up and down my client's leg, my hand makes circular friction strokes. I stand sidewards to the table with my left leg leading my right leg. Knees are bent, legs are comfortably apart and feet are stationary. No part of my body is stressed and yet I am providing the pressure required. Reverse the procedure for the left side of the client's body.

113

Avoid repetitive movements for extended periods of time. Vary the strokes you use and reduce the speed with which you do forceful, repetitive strokes to give your hands a rest.

If I've had an exceptionally hard day (numerous 250-pounders) I will use a night splint to support my wrist while I sleep. I have also used an elastic wrist bandage which I cover with a terry cloth tennis wrist band.

The wrists and hands are connected by muscles and tendons with the nerves acting as electrical messengers telling them when they are needed to move your fingers. A straight wrist will keep pressure off these muscles, tendons and nerves and will keep them relaxed, thus preventing pain.

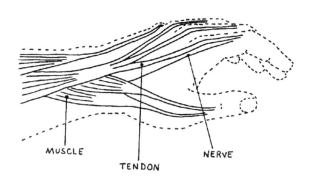

Constantly flexing your wrist forward, extending your wrist backward, or twisting your wrist to the side strains these muscles, tendons and nerves. Tension builds up in your wrists. To relieve hand and wrist tension, do the wrist flex. Place your right elbow on a desk or table, and gently bend your right hand back. Hold five seconds and repeat on the other hand. Then shake them out. I incorporate this stretch in my massage, and my clients love it.

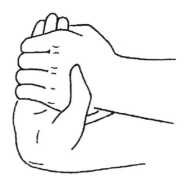

To strengthen the wrist, "work out" by squeezing a sponge or soft ball. This can be done while driving or watching TV.

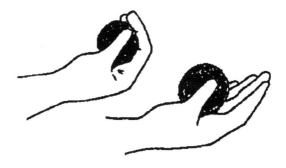

Rotate your wrists, keeping your fingers relaxed and elbows still. Start with your palms down, limp fingers hanging toward the floor. Then keeping your hands and fingers relaxed, rotate your palms up, then turn them down. Repeat five times.

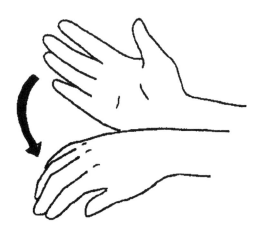

The finger fan will relax cramped fingers. Hold your hands in front of you, spread your fingers as far apart as possible. Hold for five seconds. Make a tight fist, relax,

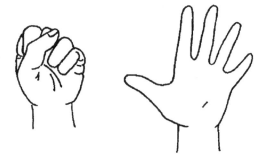

open your fingers. With hands dangling, shake your hands, up and down then sideways. Repeat this sequence three times or until the tension is gone.

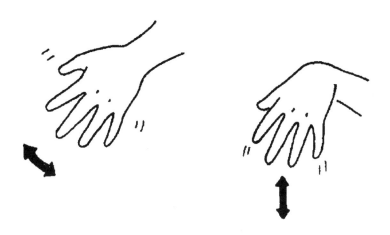

If you notice tingling, pain or numbness in the wrist, if pain wakes you up at night, if you begin to drop things, see your doctor. Shaking or massaging the wrist may work temporarily but to minimize the possibility of permanent nerve damage, *it is imperative to seek professional help as soon as possible.*

The neck (yours, that is), is another area that can suffer during a treatment. When I feel my neck start to tighten, I do head rolls as I massage. (I only do so if I'm sure my client's eyes are closed). Lower your chin to your chest, rotate your right ear to your right shoulder, bring your chin back to your chest, then lower your left

117

ear to your left shoulder. Repeat this pendulum swing until you feel relief.

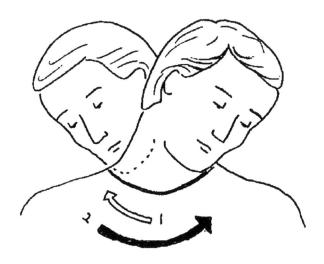

Another exercise that you may want to do in privacy is the neck glide. Though it does wonders for relieving a stiff neck, it doesn't do much for a woman's ego! Slide your head back as far as you can, keeping your head and ears level. Then slide your head forward. Do you hear all that popping and cracking? Repeat the glide three times. If you are doing it correctly, you will be creating several temporary double chins as you bring your head back, then stretching them out again as you go forward.

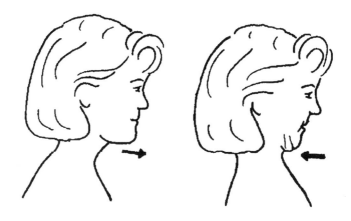

Mixing in the right stretches at the appropriate times during a massage — when you feel you need it — can give you the stamina you need to keep doing a good job for your client, from the start of his massage to the finish. You don't want your client to feel like you've "petered out" before he gets his money's worth. And it keeps you in good condition in the long run. We need to take care of ourselves if we are to take care of others.

Your upper back and shoulders can also take a beating during a massage, unless you do something yourself to prevent it. Think about your body position while massaging. Are you raising your shoulders to meet your head? If you are, you are producing your own stress while trying to alleviate your client's. Periodically, during the massage, shrug your shoulders and do an alternating shoulder roll to loosen the muscles: Pull the shoulder up, back, down and forward in a circular motion five

119

times. Roll your shoulder forward five times. Repeat five times.

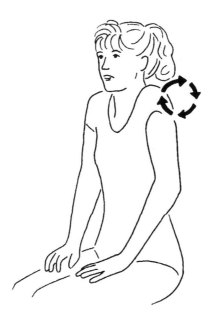

After the massage you can do more extensive stretches to keep you flexible and limber — make them as much a part of your day as brushing your teeth. First, have some fun — bring out your internal kid and "make like an airplane." Raise your arms out to the sides, elbows straight. Rev up the engines by making arm circles — slow, small circles three times forward and three times backward. This will relieve shoulder stiffness.

Now take your airplane and fly. With your arms still extended to the sides, twist your body and head to the side until a nice stretch is felt. Hold and then twist to the other side. This will loosen the upper body.

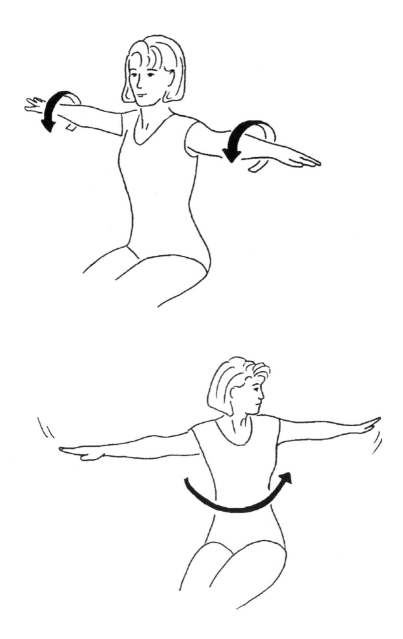

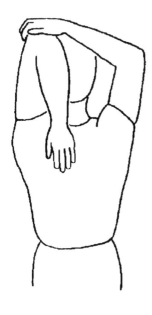

My clients tell me this stretch is very effective — and you will think so, too: For the shoulders, put the elbow behind the head and gently pull the elbow toward the center of the back until you feel a stretch. Hold for six seconds, and repeat on the other side.

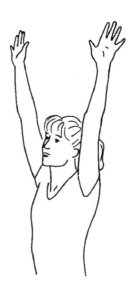

Raise your arms over your head, stretching out your fingers as you try to touch the sky. Hold for five seconds, and bring your arms down. Rest a minute. Repeat two times.

To increase the stretch in the arms, shoulders and upper back, raise your arms with your fingers interlaced and your palms facing upward. Push your arms back and up. Hold for 10 seconds.

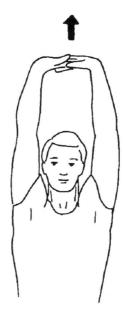

Another stretch to relieve shoulder and back tension — raise your hands to your shoulders, then push your shoulders back making sure to keep your elbows down. You can call this the "*I didn't do it!*" or the "*I give up!*" pose. Hold it for 10 seconds and repeat three times. This stretch will release muscle tension in the mid back, as well as in the upper back and shoulders. Repeat several times during the day, whenever you feel stiff or tired.

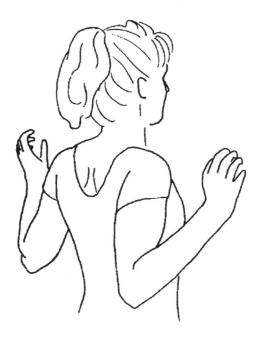

To help realign the thoracic curve and to give a stretch to the middle back, bend both elbows, swing one arm over your head and press the other arm behind your back. This is like an over-extended "running" position. Give a strong press with both arms for a maximum stretch. Hold the position for a moment, then release it and do the other side. Repeat the swings in both directions five to 10 times, as often as you feel you need it during the day.

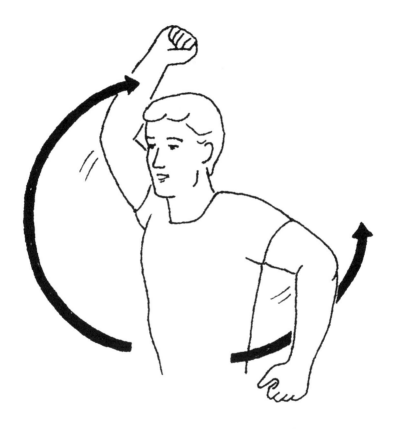

The following stretch can relieve stress in your lower back by reversing the forward bend of your spine. Stand comfortably, place your hands on the lumbar area, and *slowly* bend backward. Hold for 10 seconds. Repeat twice.

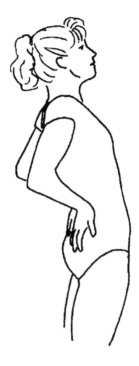

To stretch out the lower back to relieve lumbar pressure, lean forward in your chair, lower your head to your knees, touch your toes with your hands. Hold this position for a minute or two. To increase the stretch, swing your arms *under* the chair, grab the legs of the chair and pull. Make sure the chair is stable — you don't want it to slip out from under you, or to tip forward landing you on your head. Hold for 10 seconds and repeat three times.

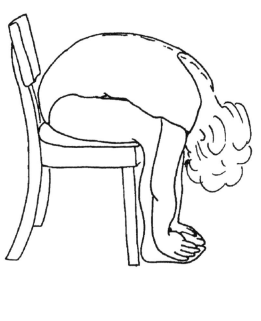

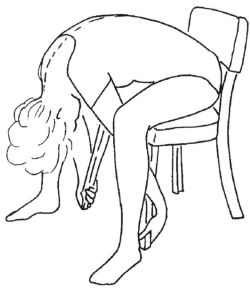

To relieve the ache in the legs caused by standing all day, lie on your back with your legs on a chair. If the edge of the chair feels uncomfortable on the back of your knees, put a small pillow under them. Rest in this position for 15 minutes.

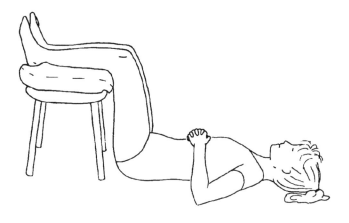

Now that you are on the floor, roll over onto all fours. Stretch one arm straight out in front of you — don't raise your head. Hold it there for a count of five. Return to all fours and repeat this stretch five times, reaching as far as you comfortably can. Switch arms and repeat, then return to the starting position, and rest. This exercise will strengthen your shoulders and upper back. Great for hard working therapists!

Return to a supine position. Slowly pull one knee to your chest while keeping your other leg and your lower back pressed against the floor. Hold for a count of five,

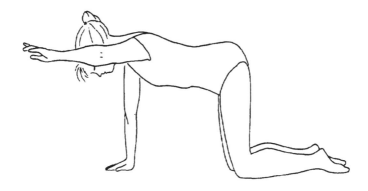

release, repeat five more times. Return the leg to the floor and repeat the pull using the other leg. Keep your feet and ankles relaxed and remember to breath! You will be giving a good stretch to the hip, lower back and buttock muscles. Your feet will also thank you if you remove them from the confines of your sneakers.

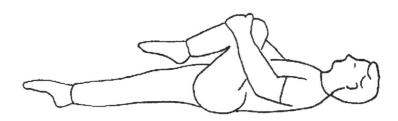

Another stretch for the lower back and buttocks is the double leg pull. While lying on your back, gently pull

129

both knees to your chest. Hold for a count of five and repeat five times.

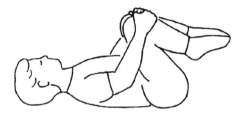

For a final all-over stretch, return to the supine position. Raise your arms over your head, point your fingers and toes, and stretch as far as you can... ahhh — doesn't that feel good! Hold for five seconds.

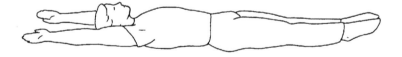

This is an excellent way to get the kinks out after a hard day. Finally, bring your arms back down to your sides, palms up, breathing quietly as you unwind in the yoga "corpse" position.

One important final suggestion: GET MASSAGED YOURSELF on a regular basis. I have heard so many therapists lament the fact that they haven't had a massage in months! This is inexcusable for a Massage Therapist. How can we expect people to put importance on what we do if we don't believe in the benefits of it for ourselves. Many of my clients ask if I get massaged and I answer with an emphatic "OF COURSE I DO!."

An inexpensive way to get your massage is to barter with another therapist. I did this in the beginning of my career. Then I found it too hard to keep even with the exchange as I sometimes needed more treatments than the person I was exchanging with. Now I pay for my massage the same as any other client. In fact, when my clients ask who massages me, and I tell them I pay to have a therapist give me treatments, they are impressed. I like what I call the "half-and-half," which has turned out to be a favorite of many of my clients as well. This is a half hour massage on the back, neck and shoulders and a half hour reflexology treatment on the feet.

So, my fellow therapist — heal thyself — GET A MAS-SAGE!

PART FIVE

Your Clients

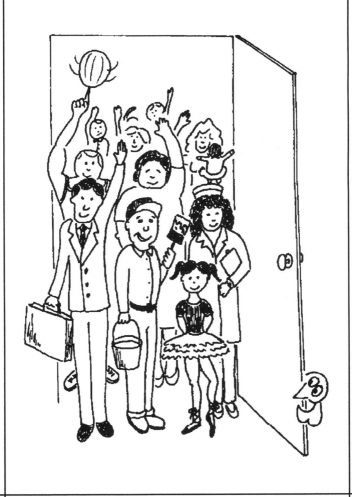

A smile never goes up in price, or down in value.

--Emmanuel

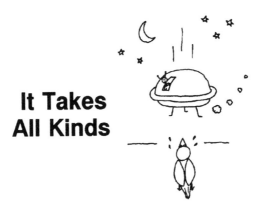

It Takes All Kinds

It stands to reason that the longer you are in business, the more people you will come in contact with. How you interact with them will either break or build your client base.

Naturally, there are as many different types of personalities as there are flowers and thorns in a garden. You may be lucky enough to have a profusion of fragrant multi-colored flowers. Then again you may find yourself getting stuck on prickly thorns.

It's the thorns that this chapter is all about.

I mean no disrespect in using the subtitles that follow; they merely describe tendencies or personality traits that fit certain clients you are likely to come across in your practice sooner or later. Knowing yourself, being comfortable with the idiosyncrasies of others and being able to empathize with their needs, will go a long way towards building trust between you and your client.

135

Next to knowing how to handle the "massage parlor" mentality, this can be the hardest part of your business because it affects your mental and emotional well-being.

This chapter was written not to taunt or titillate, but to illuminate. It is my hope that it will be received in that manner.

CLIENTS WITH HANDITIS

"Handitis" used to be my kid brother's nickname because he was always poking, slapping and hitting me.

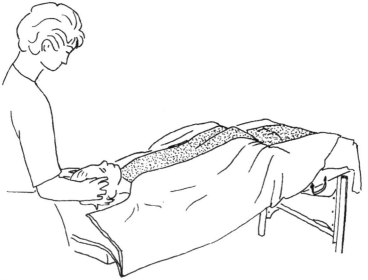

Bring the overhanging part of the flat sheet up over your client's arms when you are not working on them. It keeps drafts from creeping in — and it keeps their hands where they belong.

It now applies to clients whose hands surreptitiously seek to touch during a massage.

In PART ONE I mentioned that I use flat, flannel sheets rather than the fitted kind. I do so because the over-hang of the sheet enables me to bring it up over a client's arm and hand. This keeps a draft off them, but also, it's not so easy for them to reach out without being obvious as to their intentions.

If, in spite of all precautions, the fingers are still seeking a target, I move - either farther out from the side of the table or farther up or down the side of the table — out of reach.

If none of these ploys work, I use the direct approach and calmly say, "Please don't do that" – no hysterics, no reprimand, no explanations, just a quiet request.

THE PRIMATES

Or, what to do when your fingers get tangled in a mat of body hair?

Hairless clients are very much appreciated once you have "tangled" with the excess growth on some clients. Many men have hairy legs, some have hairy chests. Put them together with a hairy back and you have your work cut out for you. In fact, I've wished for a scissor more than once.

You have the option of not booking him again, using up your supply of oil in one session and risk having him slip off the table, or working on top of a towel. Effleurage is out of the question unless you like the frustration of constantly interrupting your stroke to unweave your fingers from the jungle.

The legs are easier to do if you use compression and small circular friction strokes. CAUTION: Unless you are practicing how to tie knots, know what you are doing! One masseur, intent on relieving spasm in the quadriceps and so out of touch with the pain he was inflicting, literally had his client tied up in knots, and actually caused the hair follicles to become inflamed and infected. His client never came back. Any wonder?

Because of the thickness of a towel, you may want to massage on top of a sheet, especially if your fingers are not too strong. I use knuckles, the heel of my hand and my finger tips. I make wide circles and I can imitate the effleurage stroke by holding the top of the sheet/towel with one hand and then making up and down movements using the pressure of knuckles or the heel of the hand.

THE AROMATICS

I had a client come to me with filthy feet and hands. Needless to say, I stayed away from them during the massage as the odor was an affront to my nostrils. I also went for my trusty bottle of Peppermint oil and mixed a few drops with the regular oil before I continued with the massage... and I did not work on the feet.

If body odor also accompanies the dirty feet, I put some Peppermint oil on a piece of cotton and lay it between the legs or on the side of the table. If you saturate the cotton and place it in a plastic baggie, it will stay aromatic and you will have it available at a moments notice. Keeping it open in the bag or on top of the bag, will prevent possible staining of your sheets. I place a towel lengthwise on my client. When massaging one buttock and leg, I am able to place the towel close to the crotch. The added covering of towel helps to mask any odor.

At the end of the massage, I ask him to take a moderately hot shower before coming for his next appointment to relax his muscles. You can be sure his condition is duly noted on his card. If he shows up again in an unkempt state, I will suggest that he book a later appointment in order that he can have an opportunity to shower before the treatment.

I give my hands a double dose of a disinfectant scrubbing. My treatment room also gets a good spraying with scented Lysol.

I have some clients who have wet hands and feet. I powder them with corn starch. (A secret nurses use to prevent BO). It not only helps with odor, but it dries the hands and feet. There are products on the market, usually baby products, which use corn starch.

As for the delicate question of vaginal odor which suggests a yeast infection, having a good rapport with your clients is invaluable. Ask after her health — has she been overly fatigued, has she noticed a vaginal discharge, has something in her life style changed which has caused her undo stress? If so, suggest a visit to her doctor for a checkup (pap smear included).

Therapists are more than mechanical dispensers of muscle tension relief. To be most effective with your treatment, your client must be your partner. There has to be trust, empathy, a giving and receiving on both sides, a caring. In simple words, a good "bedside manner." How do *you* feel when you're hurting -- physically, mentally, emotionally? What would *you* want in the form of comfort? An honest answer will go a long way towards making a mediocre "job" into a successful and rewarding career.

About halitosis: We are what we eat. If we eat garbage, we eliminate garbage and we all know how garbage stinks! Suggest a visit to a nutritionalist who will help with a healthy food plan. Notice I said, "Food Plan" not "Diet", a negative word which turns people off.

Bad breath seems to be a by-product of massage. My clients have it by the time I get to the face, which comes at the end of my massage. For the 15 minutes I work on neck, shoulders and face, I am able to turn my head, or pop a mint in my mouth.

Since my clients come to me, the air in my office is fragrant to begin with. I use: (a) a scented candle (b) aroma discs (c) incense... not necessarily at the same time! And don't forget your own personal hygiene.

THE RUMP RAISER

I can generally tell by the way a client positions himself on the table as to what kind of massage he is looking for. If one leg Is bent at a right angle and the buttock is raised, he is opening himself up for titillation.

I will straighten out the leg and will be very careful not to use any stimulating strokes. I will also be sure to stay away from the groin area. If it becomes a battle of wills — I straighten, he bends — I will shorten the length of time I work around the area and will move to the back to spend the extra time there.

When one of therapist Richard Cowan's male clients becomes aroused, he will change the place he is working and move either to the head or the feet. This has a calming, soothing effect on the client, thus allowing Richard to continue with the massage. He will also slow down his strokes if he still has work to do around the legs. Sometimes he will even eliminate the rest of the leg work and concentrate on just the feet.

If so disposed, some men will "test the waters" to see if he is amenable to "handling" their erections by saying they have gotten relief elsewhere. Richard informs them that it is not professional and offers to end the massage.

"The customer is always right" is not a hard and fast rule. You are a professional in charge of your practice. You have been trained in proper techniques and should not be intimidated into compromising your ethics.

Lesson learned — if there is any doubt in your mind about the legitimacy of a client, get the money up front. I had one client come to me who was an exceptionally difficult case to read as he came in a business suit and had given no verbal clues as to intent. Never judge a book by it's cover! Undercover detectives have tried that businessman's ploy on me also... another reason to

141

be completely ethical in all your business dealings. An easy mind sleeps soundly.

THE WIGGLER

The Wiggler is a variation of the rump raiser. He is stimulating himself by causing friction between himself and the table. In this case, I ask him to please lie still as I am not able to properly massage the muscle if it is not in a stationary position.

One of my "wigglers" took it a step further and began to pinch his nipples after I massaged his pectorals. By this time I'd had it and I told him in no uncertain terms to stop what he was doing as I pulled the towel up to his neck. He placed his hands over the towel but was careful not to move them around. Believe me, a very large notation in red was made on *his* chart... never again will his body find itself on my table!

THE FIDGET

He is so wound up that it is hard for him to lie immobile. First one leg jiggles, then the other, then both together. An arm jerks, the fingers open and close. Before you know it you find *yourself* with a twitch!

This is a good time to close your eyes and try to center yourself. I picture myself on a mountain road overlook, leaning against a white rail fence. There are white flowers swaying gently in the breeze. In the valley below there is a pristine lake. Rising up from the distant shoreline, snow-covered mountains pierce the fluffy clouds as they drift across the blue sky.

As I see and hear the song birds in my mind, I feel myself relax and I am able to continue the massage.

The calmness of my touch transfers to my client. He sighs, says "that feels good" and another client has discovered the therapeutic benefits of massage.

As a client learns to get in touch with his own body and becomes comfortable with you and your touch, the nervous twitching will subside. I can't emphasize enough about keeping yourself in the right frame of mind and developing the right attitude toward your clients. Empathy and caring pay off.

THE CONTRACTOR

The timid person contracts his muscles as a form of protection against your invading his privacy. His buttocks tighten and his hamstrings become taut. This reaction also occurs if your touch startles him. Be sure to keep your approach soft and gentle. Rest your hand quietly on the body for a second or two and then slowly rock the part that has tensed up. After you feel the muscle let go you can proceed with the massage.

Intersperse the rocking motion with your other strokes as you continue the treatment. Don't rock for too long at a time as your client will begin to feel "spacey." Stop the rocking, hold your hands still on the area, then change your stroke and continue.

Your client will also jump, giggle or contract if you happen to cause pain in the area you are working. Of course, you will back off. I do not believe in the "no pain, no gain" theory. How can you expect to release a spasm or eliminate tension if your client is working against you as he clenches his teeth and contracts his muscles against the pain you are causing him?

I can work deeply and effectively only when my client allows me to. When I hit a jumpy spot, I do effleurage, light compression and then move on to another area. I will come back and gently approach again. I lay my fingers or hand on the area to let the client know I am there. If the client contracts in anticipation of pain, I just continue to rest my hand there until I feel him relax. Then I use a little pressure. If he still contracts, I move on and come back at a later time to try again until he can accept the slight pressure. Once that happens, it's full steam ahead. Each time I back off and return, I am able to get deeper until the muscle is finally relaxed and the pain is gone.

I learned this lesson the hard — and I do mean hard — way. My first massage was almost my last massage. I was full of knotted muscles which the therapist, in her zeal, attempted to rid me of in just a half hour treatment. Tears and entreaties to go easy fell on deaf ears. It was the most painful experience I have ever had, and one I would never want to inflict on any client of mine.

My method may take a few more treatments, but when I explain the procedure my clients are more than willing to take the longer, more comfortable route, which actually turns out to be the shorter route in the long run because they trust me and will open up faster. I also make it a point not to "bleed them dry." If I'm working with chronic tension and muscle spasm, I will alternate the appointments. One time it will be a relaxing one hour treatment, the next time it will be a "working" half hour where I concentrate on the problem area.

My clients appreciate my concern for them and are very loyal. Of course, I refer out to other healthcare providers when the problem is beyond the scope of my expertise.

THE EXHIBITIONIST

There are people who are so comfortable with their own bodies that it is normal and natural to them to be uncovered in front of another person. A few types that fall into this category are sun worshipers, some dancers and underwear models.

As soon as the towel is placed over them (it would be asking too much for them to cover *themselves* with the towel provided!), the excuses start:

1. It's too hot,
2. The towel is too heavy,
3. I've never had to be covered before,

and right to the point -

4. I DON'T WANT TO BE COVERED.

Some of the solutions I've used are:

1. I put the air conditioner on and tell them that their metabolism drops when they are massaged and I have to keep them covered to prevent a chill.

2. I replace the sheet towel with a smaller, lighter towel.

3. I say that I have no control over what other therapists do in their practices but in my office my clients are covered. (This may not apply in other states but in New York it is the law).

4. Which brings me to the demand for nakedness: I use the law to my advantage so that there is no arguing back and forth. I tell them that in New York state the LAW requires that the genitals be covered. To this reply I get: "I'm not a policeman," or "I won't tell," or "No one will know."

To these entreaties I answer, *"There are no exceptions. I will not jeopardize my license, my career or my ethics. If this is not acceptable to you, then I'll understand if you don't want to come back to me."*

I will compromise with this client by using a piece of flannel the size of a hand towel which just covers the genitals. Your skill as a therapist becomes apparent as you maneuver around this loin cloth. Such a small section of material tends to slip during the rigors of some strokes. I have learned to use one hand for the technique and the other hand to hold the cloth in place. Of course, vigorous shaking strokes are out. I don't work close to the groin and I leave the area as soon as I can. So what if this isn't one of your better massages... most of these people are more interested in their fantasy then they are in your technique.

When I was approached with complaints of a "groin pull," I laughed to myself — another ploy, I thought. However, it is a legitimate complaint with competitive athletes.

I question my client closely to ascertain the cause of the problem and then I decide the course of my treatment. My small piece of material allows me to get in close to the origin of the quads and still keep my client covered. I also use the cloth to move the genitals out of the way without touching skin.

You can be sure that only someone with a legitimate groin pull will subject himself to this treatment a second time, because it can be very painful. Everyone else seems to make a miraculous recovery!

I have some very creative clients. When I ask if they are ready for me, they say yes. When I enter the room they are standing, facing me with nothing on but a big grin. They get no reaction from me as I ask them to lay on the table face down.

So, stand your ground. The good word gets around as well as the bad.

THE CLIENT WHO TALKS, AND TALKS, AND TALKS...

I feel a kinship with this person. I am not one who is comfortable with the "pregnant pause." I feel compelled to fill every gap in conversation, and more often than not, I fill it with my foot.

147

One lady kept repeating, "I'm so embarrassed, I'm so embarrassed — I've never had a massage before." Ladies such as this generally keep their bras on. I then have to go through the gyrations of keeping her covered while she struggles out of her garment. After she settles down, out pours the sad tale of what caused her current pain.

This purging is as necessary to the healing process as is the educated touch of your hands. We are the lay person's unofficial psychologist. We don't prescribe or diagnose, but we are there for them. We are a sounding board, a willing ear.

One client sat with me for 15 minutes just unburdening herself. At the end she heaved a relieved sigh, gave me a hug and said, "I needed you to listen to me today even more than I needed your healing hands — thank you."

Can anyone put a price tag on such a relationship? I for one feel blessed and grateful that I have been given the gift of caring.

Another client was so shy that she lay on the table clad in pantyhose and a latex one-piece bathing suit. Talk about having your work cut out for you! I was able to coax her to lower the top of the suit and then explained the difficulty involved in trying to massage through such attire. After a few "getting to know me" sessions she felt comfortable enough with just the towel covering her. Trust on her part, understanding on mine.

As we begin to build a rapport with each other, I explain the treatment process in detail — how allowing themselves to become enmeshed in the experience will produce quicker relaxation. Many people do not know how to get in touch with themselves. Your office can be their classroom.

I use environmental water tapes because water has healing qualities. Depending on which tape I am using, I start them off with an appropriate picture: "We are on a sailboat; I'm going to Tahiti — you go wherever you'd like to be." Or, "I'm sitting by a babbling stream with cool water tickling my toes as it flows over my feet."

After their first nervously gabby session, I ask them to silently go along with the sensations they are experiencing. Certainly they can speak to me if I should hit a sore spot or if they need to express a thought. I know they're "getting with the program" by the number of sighs they utter. I try to make them more aware of what they are feeling rather than what I am doing.

At the end of the treatment, the women say they feel like melted butter. As for the men, I generally have to wake them up.

To perfect your technique and your contact with your client try massaging to light classical music. Change your tempo and the type of stroke to blend with the music. Practice on a willing friend first in order to make your hand transitions smooth. You'll find you will truly be "with" your client. The music flows to your ears, the rhythm transfers to your hands; you hands "play" the tune on your client's body. You and your client have become one through the sound and the touch. And the healing circle is complete, not only for the client but for you as well. I find this an excellent technique to use when I am feeling tired. I become so caught up with the music that I too am in a state of euphoria that soothes my psyche as well as my client's.

THE SHY SHARON/MODEST MYRTLE

Michael J. Aronoff, a therapist in Great Neck, NY, says that one of the biggest obstacles he had to overcome was the reluctance some women had to try massage given by a man. There were those who had never had a massage at all, and were shy about disrobing for *anyone*.

A tip he would like to share which went a long way to building trust between his clients and himself was careful draping during the treatment. He also keeps the room warm and plays soft music.

Louis Augier, another New York therapist, shares his practice with a female. While not the case in New York, some states deem it illegal to practice cross-gender massage. Louis and his partner, Robin, therefore felt they could offer the public this added option by working together.

Louis recalls a phone conversation with a female who asked if a man or a woman would be doing the massage. When told it would be a male, the client expressed concern, saying she had never been massaged by a man before. Lou suggested that she come into the office to meet with him so that he could dispel her fears. When she realized Lou was the therapist, she remarked that he sounded like a nice enough person and booked her appointment then and there. She has since become a steady client.

Lou believes that peoples' objections are based on deep seated feeling and should be accepted as such — neither right nor wrong, simply as feelings. Once an objection to a male therapist is expressed as a feeling and nothing more, then it must be respected. He makes every attempt possible to meet personally with the client and he goes over the massage procedure very thoroughly, especially if it is a first time massage.

Lou employs a technique whereby he non-threateningly makes physical contact with his client. While explaining Oriental Massage, he politely asks for her arm so he can demonstrate the coursing of the long meridian to her. This not only affords her a hands-on demo of Amma Therapy, but it also allows a direct exchange of their energies, which is his motive.

He finds that taking the time to answer all their questions and explaining procedure and draping while maintaining good eye contact, has made a significant difference in the amount of women who have changed their original opinion and now permit him to massage them.

His greatest satisfaction comes when a female client grasps his hand and genuinely thanks him for explaining all that he did about massage. Lou's advice is to reach out and with caring and understanding, take the time to educate wherever and whenever you can.

For therapist Scott Meyers, who works at a Holistic Center, his "modest Myrtle" was a "Michael." One of his female clients bought a gift certificate for her boyfriend, but when they arrived at the Center and the man realized it was Scott who would be massaging him, he froze. In order to put him at ease, Scott suggested that the woman stay in the room during the treatment. Scott kept speaking to the woman, showing her what he was doing and why. The man's eyes may have been closed, but his ears were taking in all that was being said. Before long the client began to relax enough so that Scott felt he was able to give him a credible treatment.

Rip Stahura, a competitive power lifter as well as a massage therapist, found that his problem was not so much with his clients as with his "significant other." His lady objected to him working on other women. Rip found that in order to keep the peace he had to cut down his practice by as much as 50 percent.

As he uses Amma in his practice, he explains the procedure to his female clients beforehand so that they are prepared for his touch when he has to work the intercostals. He has also found that when people are looking for the right treatment for their particular problem, they don't care if the therapist is male or female. They just want the right modality to get the job done.

If you are working with a chiropractor or medical team, the involvement of the other professionals can sometimes ease clients' concerns.

For example, therapist Thomas Redes began his practice working for three different chiropractic groups. At only one did he experience any reluctance on the part of patients to being massaged by him because he was a male, a problem he felt stemmed from the fact that he was filling in for the regular therapist, who was female. The patients, mostly female, expressed their reluctance to the chiropractor, who informed Tom. A conference was set up with the doctor, individual patient, and Tom, and the situation was resolved to the satisfaction of all concerned.

Tom also works in a health and racquetball club, where he found the reticence is on the part of some of the men. Some male clients say they would not want a man to work on them. This comment is usually said with an accompanying snicker or leer, conveying a homophobic point of view, and a fear of what others might think of them.

Some women express reluctance toward a male therapist from a sexist/safety viewpoint — they feel that if they are alone with a man, something sexual must transpire. Other women express concern about exposing their cellulite, or some other aspect of a less-than-perfect body, to a man's eyes. (Would that we were ALL in perfect shape!).

When Tom has these attitudes relayed to him, he finds that spending time talking with the person about their apprehensions helps. When there are concerns like these, he has found that the women seem more open than the men to at least trying a session with a male therapist.

Most people are open to massage whether the therapist is male or female. It is the people who have a preconceived "massage parlor" view of massage who express fear and concern. Tom has found that experiences of this kind represent only a small percentage of his clientele, however.

THE WEEPING WILLOW

I must confess to knowing this type first hand. It's me. It must have been "one of those days," or else I was more needy than even I knew. At any rate, right in the middle of an Amma treatment, I burst into tears and just couldn't stop the flow.

The therapist, in his desire to help me, started to give me all kinds of instructions... breath deeply, think of something pleasant, relax, etc. I was embarrassed and tried my darndest to stem the tide, which only succeeded in giving me a pain in my stomach. The purging tears were never allowed to finish the job and I felt drained and uneasy.

From that experience I learned to allow my client to let go without censure, without comment, without making a big thing out of it. What I do is whisper, "It's okay," and I will lay my hands quietly on his shoulder for a few seconds. Then I will gently stroke his face, murmuring softly, "It's okay, it's okay." Gradually the anguish passes, the purge has been fully completed, and the massage continues without further incident.

I had a client who was newly divorced. The trauma of the separation surfaced during the massage and he began to cry uncontrollably. He asked me to hold him, which I did, cradling him in my arms and rocking him back and forth the way a mother would do with a hurt child. After a while he quieted down, sighed, smiled at me and said "thank you." No further mention was made of the episode and the session went on as though nothing unusual had happened.

THE CHRONIC LATE-COMER/NO-SHOW

If you are, as I am, one of those "show up before time" people, you know how distressing it can be to have your nicely scheduled appointment book start to look like a pre-schooler's scratch pad.

Unfortunately, most of us don't have the overflow practice many doctors have and therefore can't over-book. Nor do many of us have ample waiting room space where clients can cool their heels while waiting to be received into the inner sanctuary.

I have made it a practice, in my social life, to wait up to a half hour for friends who aren't as compulsive about time commitments as I am. I have carried that policy over in my business. I allow 15 minutes to a half hour between appointments. This prevents a time crunch if someone is late, or if someone is early. If, praise be, everything is running on time, I have 15-to-30-minutes to rest and recoup my energy.

If a client is so late as to encroach on another's appointment, they know that their time is reduced in proportion to the time they have overstepped the bounds.

As for "No-Shows," here is where I overbook. These appointments are made by "just looking" types who are window shopping for the best price, or they are those characters looking for the wrong kind of "relief."

Though I have been able to screen out most of them over the phone, they are becoming more educated than the legitimate population. They know how I will reply to their queries and they have called enough therapists to know how to answer my questions. They know that we know what they *really* want to know: *"Do you do full body massage?"*

Of course we do. But what they are really asking is if we give "release." One smart-alec asked that if I massaged all the muscles why did I leave out the penis which he considered a very important muscle that gave him a lot of stress!

At one time emphasis was put on the word FULL. When they realized I knew what the emphasis implied, they eliminated that tactic but still asked the same question. My answer is, "Yes I do, *with the exception of the genitals.*" This is where they get cute — they deny that was what they had in mind (ha, ha) and then 'they make a day appointment. (Suspect right there. Don't they work?).

If they want an evening appointment, I schedule them as early after work as they can get to me. No late nights for new clients. Then I book them on the half hour, say 6:30 p.m. If I get a call from a regular client for 6 p.m. I take it. The regular comes from 6 to 7. *If* the new client does arrive at 6:30, a note on the door informs him that I'm running late and to please wait. I leave the Client Information Card and the Health Questionnaire for him to fill out while he waits. There are also a few magazines to read. At most he has a half hour to wait.

If he doesn't show, I haven't lost an hour. If he had booked a one-hour treatment, the next appointment I would make would be for 7:30, and I have a half hour to rest. I would try to make the 7:30 appointment for a half-hour treatment, though, so that if he *did* come, but I didn't take him until 7 (after my regular client), I would be finished with him by 8, and the half-hour booking would then get me back on schedule.

I try to get a phone number from new clients, and ask for both a work and a home number. The next day I call the number to confirm that it is indeed his number. If it turns out to be bogus, the appointment is erased (it was written in pencil until confirmed), and my hour is once again open.

All this may sound confusing and time consuming, but it will save a lot of grief in the long run.

Don't believe everything your clients tell you while they are on the table, and don't be coerced into doing anything that will compromise your sense of ethics. Amnesia develops as soon as they get off the table!

There have been occasions when I have had to emphatically refuse clients' requests. Only then will they finally believe that I mean what I say, and begrudgingly pay me the supreme compliment — "I know, you're a professional!"

Isn't that what it's all about?

157

PART SIX

The Nitty Gritty

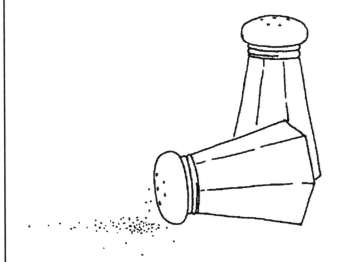

Humor is the hole that lets
sawdust out of a stuffed shirt.

--Unknown

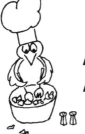

A Little of This, A Bit of That...

What follows are pieces of advice, most of which were learned the hard way. I wish I had the sense to know about them *before* I started practicing. Most of them make very good sense when you think about them, it's just that, we don't think of them. Forewarned is forearmed.

Caesar Salads, Heads and Tales Unless you are working in a health club or spa where there are showers, it is a good idea *NOT* to make a Caesar Salad out of your client. I've had several people complain about therapists who use too much oil. Remember, they have to put their clothes back on. Besides, if you are using too much lubricant you aren't giving a good massage because you can't get in deep if you are slipping and sliding all over the place.

Another tip when working on the head — remember, you are giving a massage, not a shampoo. If a client is going out in public after leaving your establishment, they don't want to look like a punk rocker with their hair standing on end because you used too much oil, and massaged their hair instead of their scalp.

Stay away from the head altogether if your client, man or woman, comes in with hair spray welding each strand together. You can be *sure* they do not want to be messed up. It's difficult to restyle teased hair that has been given an oil bath. I do very little head work in this situation and I *always* smooth the hair back into place as best I can.

Be on the lookout for men wearing hairpieces. One client neglected to inform me of his toupee, so you can imagine my surprise when my fingers met the mesh base. Needless to say, I left the area immediately to work elsewhere.

Another client, with a dry sense of humor, said he would remove his "rug" if I had some double-sided tape he could use to replace it.

I do not add oil to my hands when working on the face. In fact, I wipe my hands off before starting the face massage. Most people have enough natural oils without your having to add more. In fact, ladies who come in with a face made up for a night on the town do not want their cosmetics disturbed. If you do a face massage and use special oils for that purpose, or if your clients come in with squeaky clean faces, then you needn't be concerned.

I do, however, use Peppermint Oil when working on the forehead. It not only does wonders for a headache, but it goes a long way in relaxing your client.

162

Therapist Joe Salerno is careful not to touch the face if his client is wearing make-up. He found that no matter how careful he was while working around the neck, he still got some oil on his client's hair. Now he uses skin conditioner exclusively in his massages.

Hot oils Several of my clients like hot oil for their massages. I recycled an old electric baby bottle warmer. A word of caution, though — the warmer worked so well that I burned my hands when I took out the bottle of oil. Now I wrap the bottle in a face cloth which helps keep the oil warm, and my hands cool.

One Good Turn... When you ask your clients to turn over, do they clutch at the towel? Women are great at doing this. Some men, on the other hand, just love to have the towel "slip." Instead of raising the towel above the body as they turn, I keep it low and in contact with their skin, not up in the air. This keeps them warm and leaves them with their modesty uncompromised.

Towel Tip Most of the time I work on top of the towel when working from the solar plexus to the abdominals. I hold the top edge with one hand to keep it in place while massaging with the other hand. At one time I drew the towel down to the pelvic area until I noticed that occasionally I was coming in contact with pre-ejaculation fluid. Leaving the male client toweled prevents this. When I massage a man's chest I fold the towel down to just below the breast bone to work the intercostals and pectorals. For women I slip one hand under the towel (working from the head down) to do the intercostals.

Home Alone If you're working out of your home or apartment, especially if you are a single woman, give the appearance that someone else beside yourself resides with you.

I had a gentleman friend who smoked a pipe. I asked him for one of his old corn cobs and left it, with some ashes, in the ash tray in a prominent place in my living room.

If you are in a studio apartment, buy a studio bed instead of a regular bed so there is no intimate connotation to what you are doing.

Display pictures of a boyfriend, husband, children (borrow some of your friends' relatives if you have none of your own). Wear a wedding ring or any kind of costume jewelry that would give the impression that you're married. If you have a new client and you will be working late, have a friend (preferably male) call your answering machine to say that he is on his way home. Have a girlfriend call to say she'll be stopping by for a cup of coffee. Make the call an actuality so that your story will have credibility.

When I first began my career, I worked out of my one-bedroom apartment. To provide necessary privacy in limited quarters, I divided my living room by hanging roll-up bamboo shades from the ceiling. In the event a couple came together, one person had a comfortable seating area in the living room while the other had the privacy of the partitioned section. When I had no clients I rolled up the shades to open up the room and to allow the light and sunshine to brighten up the area.

164

Mint Condition I've previously mentioned breath mints. Have a small dish into which you can empty a package of *Dynamints* or *Tic Tacs,* and place it on the side table within reach for when you work on the head, neck and shoulders.

Remember we talked about clients who have halitosis. Don't think you are immune just because you are the practitioner. At the end of my massage I lean close and whisper, "When you're ready, get up slowly so that you don't get dizzy." This let's them know that the massage is over and that I'm breaking contact. After giving my all for an hour, I don't want to risk negating the treatment by breathing garlic in a client's face! One asked me for a mint himself, saying that was a very nice service to provide.

The mints, along with a glass of water, keep your mouth moist as you work.

Use A Bolster Place it under the knees when the client lies on his back. This makes for easy draping of the towel in the groin area, it eases pressure on the spine, it provides a prop for my oil, and it allows me to work the origin of the quadriceps without disturbing the genitals. Keep your hands moving and don't linger here unnecessarily... and for heaven's sake, don't tell a man who is embarrassed over his involuntary erection to have his wife take care of his needs before he comes for a massage!

Use A Flat Sheet It works better than a fitted one on the table because it allows me to flip one side of it over my client's body to keep them warm, to keep their hands from touching me, and to keep the oil on their body from rubbing off on my clothing.

Also, the flat sheet hangs down over the sides of the table, hiding the hamper I keep underneath. I can fold the end section over the feet, again, to keep the heat in and to remind me *not* to massage the feet of a client with ticklish soles.

I have several clients going through separations or divorces. To provide them with a warm feeling of safety and security, I wrap them in a cocoon of sheet and towel (ever try doing that with a fitted sheet?). The sheet is brought up from the side of the table and tucked under the shoulder. When I am massaged, I like this tucking because it keeps air from getting under the towel and chilling me.

Cuts and Hangnails If you've ever been bothered by them, you know the pain involved with trying to give a massage with them. I use "Nu Skin" or "Skin Shield," which are liquid bandages. They are antiseptic, water-proof, flexible, and they can be bought in a drug store.

When Inspiration Strikes... If you are anything like me, you get ideas at the most inappropriate times, when pad and pencil are nowhere in sight, or in the middle of a massage. In this case, I use memory pegs to remind me of my "terrific thought."

For example, I wanted to write about the Turtle and the Hare, make an insertion in this chapter ("Nitty Gritty"), and develop an idea I had for Playdoh. T N P became the memory pegs for Turtle, Nitty Gritty, and

Playdoh. As I kept repeating the letters over and over, they became a part of the rhythm of my massage and I was able to recall my thoughts later.

I even wake up in the middle of the night with a brain storm. Without opening my eyes I reach for the pad and pencil I keep by the bed, and jot the thought down. Of course the handwriting leaves much to be desired and I sometimes run off the page, but enough is saved to jog my memory in the morning. A small flashlight alongside the pad and pencil can be a great help. Or have a tape recorder at bed side — a simple flip of the switch will save your thought.

Do your priceless gems attack in the midst of your morning shower? An underwater tablet and writing implement will keep that thought from going down the drain. If you don't have a scuba store near you where they sell such things, then brave the chillies of the bathroom to reach outside the shower curtain for your trusty pad and pencil. Yes, my writing tools are right there with the powder, deodorant, hair spray...

The Gift of Massage In my treatment room I have a sign which reminds my clients that Gift Certificates are available. During the holidays I put up a Santa Claus poster (very colorful and handmade) in a prominent spot that can't be missed as they dress and undress for their massage. Sticking out of Santa's pack are Gift Certificates instead of toys.

First Timers Actual table time for a client's first visit is 45 to 50 minutes. The first part of the hour is spent filling in client history forms and getting acquainted.

Taking time to be personable is *not* short-changing your client.

Nurturing Loyalty Anything (within reason and legal!) you can do that will enable you to stand out in the crowd will go a long way to encourage client loyalty. When I sell Gift Certificates I offer the buyer a choice of stickers to personalize their gift even more. I have heart stickers, happy face stickers, stickers that say Happy Birthday, Congratulations and Happy Anniversary. They are very pleased with my thoughtfulness and have a great time deciding which sticker to use and where to put it.

Be Whole to Make Whole Keep in mind *your* state of mind. If you are agitated, the massage will feel like a roller coaster ride to your client. If you are serene the massage will take on the peaceful nature of a tranquil canoe ride on a mountain lake.

Massage is a medley of sensations: the aroma of scented candles or incense, the sound of environmental tapes, the security of low lighting, the warmth of flannel sheets on the skin and finally, the soothing, caring touch of my hands.

Cradle Covers Remember my suggestion for the loin cloth? I made good use of the remainder of the flannel by making covers for the table headrest. I had tried paper towels, face cloths, no cloths and finally, with the help of my daughter-in-law's sewing expertise, my problem was solved. She measured an oval larger than one of the headrest pillows, make a casing and inserted very narrow elastic to make it fit.

Once a pattern was made it was simple to make sets of three. I had plenty of material left to give me a good supply of covers which are changed as routinely as my sheets.

These covers also work beautifully with the on-site chair and the massage mate.

Protect Your Knees I found that I was making dents in my housemaid's knees every time I rested them against the wooden end brace at the head of my table. A trip to the local fabric store yielded a length of foam padding which I used to wrap the cross piece. I also wrapped the wood end brace at the foot of my table, which saved my knees when I sat to do reflexology.

Giveaways A word about handouts — whenever a new client fills out the health questionnaire, he gets my card and a pen imprinted with my name and phone number to keep. I have had people tell me they lost my card but were able to contact me because they kept my pen.

I had key chains made with a soft rubber foot which I passed out at any business function I went to, along with my card. I became known as the "Foot Lady" to my fellow business associates.

It does pay to advertise uniquely in order to make yourself stand out and be remembered.

In keeping with my reflexology business, I had vanity plates made which read, "HAPIFEET." Another memory peg was established and I became known by that name.

Even when I gave up those plates, acquaintances still called me by that handle... and I am remembered.

Many Happy Returns... A final tip: Please return your phone calls. I know therapists use their answering machines to screen calls because of the unsavory element who gravitates to massage. Many female therapists eliminate male clients unless they are recommended. This could curtail your business.

Try to perfect your telephone screening technique. My telephone listing appears close to the bottom of the column because my company name begins with "T." Since I am always curious as to where my business comes from, I ask why I was called instead of those above my listing. Having a corporate name may have something to do with it, but more often than not I am told I was the *only one* on the list who had returned their call!

Common courtesy can pay off.

PART SEVEN

Added Income

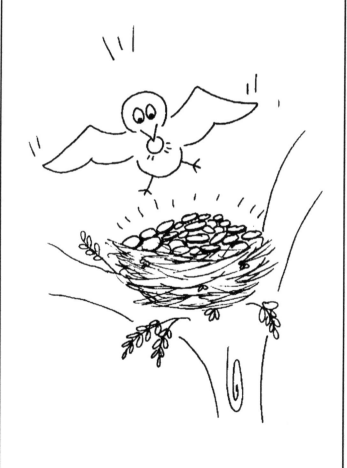

Everything comes to him
who hustles while he waits.

--Thomas Edison

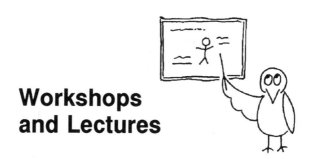

Workshops and Lectures

This book is the outgrowth of workshops I gave on "So You Want To Make Money in Your Chosen Profession."

Workshops differ from lectures in that they are generally smaller, more intimate gatherings of people who are interested in a specific subject who have come to interact with the presenter. Workshops tend to have a life of their own.

Lectures usually have a more formal format and involve larger audiences. Whereas the time allotted for a lecture may have to be strictly adhered to, workshops tend to just flow along with the energy of the group.

Reimbursement for a lecture is generally a predetermined figure, whether 50 or 150 show up. With workshops, each person is charged a certain amount. Remember that there are expenses that need to be considered when setting your price: Are you renting space? Are you providing handouts? How much do you want to earn an hour? Are you paying to advertise the event?

A good idea to prod sign-ups is to offer a discount (here I go again!) for early registration. A free gift is also an incentive to encourage interest in your class. Stressdots fit the bill very nicely as a give-away. Everyone likes a bargain.

Getting on the lecture circuit isn't all that hard. Getting paid is another story. Everyone has to pay their dues, so look on "freebies" as a learning/perfecting process. You are becoming known as an expert in your field, you are becoming more comfortable speaking before groups, you are also getting exposure and free publicity.

Be your own PR person. This is the place where it's okay to blow your own horn, and if you don't you're losing out on a golden opportunity. I send out a press release complete with a black and white photo to my area newspaper after each presentation. You'd be surprised how often people will come up to you to say they saw your picture in the paper. People like to be associated with "celebrities."

Organizations are always looking for guest speakers. For service organizations like Kiwanis, Rotary, Lions, you speak for 15 to 20 minutes. As you get proficient in your subject you'll find it harder to speak for a short time because you will have so much information to share — and if you let it be known that you have much more to say but that you don't want to take up their valuable time, you can be sure you will be asked back. Command performances look great on your resume.

The secret to making a successful talk is to remember the three S's:

Keep it Short,
Keep it Simple, and
Sit down.

Inform your audience. Involve your listeners. Entertain them. And have fun yourself. It's contagious!

A word of caution, however: Know your audience. I spoke at my Kiwanis Club on "Surviving Stress Sensibly." An informative subject for business people, I thought. To involve them I placed tennis balls on the tables, which I use to show how to relieve stress in the shoulders. Wrong move. They entertained themselves by *throwing the balls at each other* instead of using them the way I had intended!

Balls were flying everywhere — I was grateful they were not aimed at me. I waited until they were finished, but I knew I had lost them along with the tennis balls, so I kept it *short* and I *sat down.*

In contrast, I spoke before a group of 150 people using the same speech. This time I threw about six balls into the audience without a problem. If the balls are not returned to me, I am not concerned because I write my name and telephone number with magic marker on each one — free advertising!

You will be surprised at how fast your name will be circulated once you speak at a few functions. A free meal, a chance to hand out your cards, confidence and experience gained, are all non-monetary pluses. Add the thrust of a press release with your picture and pretty soon you are known as an expert. The phone will ring, and one day you will be asked what your speaking fee is. Now you are not only an expert but a professional speaker as well.

I started out charging $50 to a group of university students because I knew money was tight for them. The fun we all had more than made up for the small fee. They were so appreciative that I received a very nice thank you note, which was added to my publicity file.

I set my rate scale according to the circumstances of the engagement—where it is held (do I have to travel?), the number of people attending, the length of the talk. As your popularity increases and the demand for what you have to offer grows, so will the fee that you can charge.

If you are interested in pursuing this avenue of income, an excellent book to read is <u>Speak and Grow Rich</u> by Dottie Walters. She takes you by the hand and step-by-step covers all the pros and cons of this very lucrative business.

Writing is akin to speaking. We therapists have a responsibility to educate the public, and what better platform than the printed word?

I am a member of my local Chamber of Commerce (a good business move). A local paper works closely with the Chamber reporting news of the town. I have worked out an arrangement with the publishers whereby I pay for an ad every other month, and I can submit an article on health-related subjects, *with my by-line*, every month. I keep track of where people hear about me, and this vehicle has proven very lucrative.

Action TNT:
Today, Not Tomorrow.

--Unknown

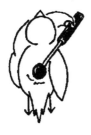

Bongers, Stressdots and Tapes

Bongers are nothing more than a rubber ball attached to a flexible handle, but do they ever do a job on tense muscles!

I keep a bonger in my car and pass the time waiting at red lights and in traffic jams, beating out the muscle tension in my shoulders. My bonging does double duty. It not only relieves my stress, it also brings a smile to the face of the driver next to me.

I keep bongers in my office. No one can resist asking what they are. When I tell them they are human meat tenderizers and show them how to reduce muscle tension and stimulate circulation between visits, I make a sale. I also mention their value as a fun gift for that person who has everything.

When you order bongers (see APPENDIX on how to order bongers and stressdots), they come packaged two in a box. I sell them singly, and to make them more appealing I encase the ball in a plastic wrap, draw a happy face on it and tie the plastic with colorful ribbon.

179

I attach an instruction booklet to the ribbon to make sure the bongerer knows *not* to bong the kidneys.

I also bring bongers to any event where I am doing massage. I not only bonger my client to demonstrate the procedure, but I also allow those waiting in line to try bongering while they wait. A friend is available to take names and addresses of anyone interested in buying them.

I was at a meeting of the National Speakers Association (an excellent organization, by the way, to learn how to perfect your speaking talents — for information write to them at 3877 N. 7th St., #350, Phoenix, AZ 85014). Networking tables were set up for the members to display their cards, brochures, flyers, etc. I brought my bongers along, demonstrated, and sold every one.

Stressdots

Stressdots are circles of micro-encapsulated liquid crystal that records the changes in peripheral skin temperature by changing to one of seven colors. They are worn on the hand and will remain for up to 48 hours of continual monitoring.

The change in color alerts you to changes in blood flow which occurs during a stressful situation. With this awareness of when stress is on the rise, a person can apply a relaxation exercise "on the spot" to interrupt the cycle.

I put a dot on my clients when they come for their appointments. The dot is generally amber or olive colored, reflecting their stressful state of mind. I even put one on my own hand. When the massage is completed we look at the dots again. Invariably they have changed to turquoise or blue, indicating relaxation. Even after working for an hour, my dot has changed to blue. If it doesn't, I know it's time to take stock of what's happening in my own life. It is a good biofeedback method which keeps me on target with my own health program. Remember, "Therapist Heal Thyself."

I usually give my clients a few dots to use at home in order to get them started on their awareness program. When they come for their next treatment, they buy packets of dots for themselves and for their friends and relatives.

I hand out stressdots when I give lectures on Stress Management. Everyone is curious about them. This keeps your audience attentive while they wait to find out what they are all about.

Bongers and stressdots make great holiday or birthday gifts, and along with gift certificates are thoughtful *gifts of health.*

Tapes

As far as tapes are concerned, you may want to forgo this expense until you are comfortable with your speaking engagements.

Tapes have the advantage of allowing your audience to "take you home with them." Most of what we hear in a lecture is forgotten by the time we get home, and note

181

taking can be tedious. I find that I am so concerned with writing everything down that I miss a good part of what is going on anyway. Knowing I can buy a tape to refresh my memory at my leisure helps me to concentrate on the speaker's delivery and the content of his talk.

For example, I attended an all-day seminar on Stress Management. The speaker was very good; she had handouts and a workbook for us to fill in as we followed along with her talk. I noticed that in the morning she wore high heels, but at the end of the morning break she had changed to shoes with more comfortable heels. And then it happened. During the afternoon session she kicked off her shoes and continued her presentation in her stocking feet.

What was my lasting impression of that day? You're right. A nice lady standing on the platform in her stocking feet. (Remember the chapter on being professional?).

A big advantage to making tapes is that you can retape as often as you like until you get it right. Taping gives you an opportunity to hear how you sound to others and to correct speech patterns, pitch or tonal quality which could grate on the ears of your listeners.

Taking a booth at Health Fairs is another outlet for selling your tapes. You can speak on any number of health-related subjects which is a good tie-in for advertising your expertise as a massage therapist.

There are any number of audiotape production companies in the phone book to check out when you are ready to go this route. If you know any band groups, ask where they get their demos made.

And finally, still looking for ways to add to your income? WRITE A BOOK!

People rarely succeed at anything unless they have fun doing it.

--Author unknown

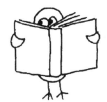

Epilogue

Remember you are a human computer — what you think is what you get. A positive thought and a negative thought cannot occupy the same space at the same time. What are the negative thoughts that are taking up valuable, productive "bytes" in your human computer?

Only you know your personal inhibitors. Is it fear of not having a steady income? Is it confusion as to which direction your practice should take? Is it anxiety about establishing your reputation as a credible therapist? Is it self-pity because you feel so isolated in your career?

Whatever your personal inhibitors are, write them down. Be honest.

Now that you have written down your negatives and have looked at what immobilizes you, you can face them head-on. Once you have faced them, you can now erase them. Sit comfortably in a chair, close your eyes, see your inhibitors, and let them go. Stuff each one into a balloon and watch it float away until it is no longer visible.

Now visualize a huge hot air balloon firmly anchored to the ground. With a brush, paint a constructive positive on it in a bright fluorescent color. Stand back and let the brilliant, sparkling word burn itself into your consciousness. If you do not replace the negative immediately with a positive, another negative might fill the void.

The process — called the Mitchell Technique — can be summed up as the IFER PROCEDURE:

I dentify it
F ace it
E rase it
R eplace it

If you set your goals and work your plan, but do not retain a positive mental outlook, then all will have been in vain. Every man is the architect of his own fortune.

Someone once said, "Freedom is doing what you like. Happiness is liking what you do." We have chosen a very special, a wonderful, healing profession. What we do is touch lives. There's so much to like about what we do, let's not allow negatives to side-track or hinder us. Will Rogers said, "Even if you're on the right track, you'll get run over if you just sit there."

I wish you the joy of a job well done. I wish you the pleasure of wonderful clients. And above all, I wish you the gratification of knowing that, as a massage therapist, you have touched your fellow human beings in a positive, caring manner.

Good fortune.

Appendix

Appendix

A collection of suppliers, books and resources that should prove valuable to every massage therapist. These items, books and organizations are only a small sample of what is available.

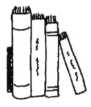 BOOKS — ON BUSINESS

Business Mastery, by Cherie Sohnen-Moe
Sohnen-Moe Associates
3906 W. Ina Road #200-3487
Tucson, AZ 85741
(602) 744-0094

The Business of Massage, by Maryann Capó
Ten Plus Ten
469 Hawkins Avenue
Lake Ronkonkoma, NY 11779
(516) 585-5691

Business Savvy
Health Action
19 East Mission #102
Santa Barbara, CA 93101

The Insurance Reimbursement Manual, by Christine Rosche
Bodytherapy Business Institute
10441 Pharlap Drive
Cupertino, CA 95014

Massage & Bodywork Resource Guide, by Robert Calvert, with Noel Abildgaard
Noah Publishing Company
PO Box 1500
Davis, CA 95617

Record Keeping for Massage Professionals and
Your Successful Massage-Bodywork Practice, by Jefferson Saunders, LMT
c/o N.E.I. Publishing and Marketing
PO Box 20445
Seattle, WA 98102-1445
(206) 329-3566

Speak and Grow Rich, by Dottie Walters

Tax Tips for the Self-Employed Bodyworker, by Paul A. Kirchhoff, MA, LMT, and Paul L. Harold, MBA, CPA
Health Management Group
3742 Arelia Drive North
Delray Beach, FL 33445
(407) 393-1139

190

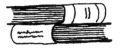 BOOKS — ON MASSAGE AND HEALTH

The following books are excellent resources, and are generally available, unless otherwise noted.

Are You Tense?, by Ben Benjamin

Feet First, A Guide to Foot Reflexology, by Laura Norman

Hands-On Healing, published by Prevention Magazine

The Healing Power of Humor, by Allen Klein

Ice Therapy—Understanding Its Application, by Harold Packman (PO Box 3, Whitestone, NY 11357)

Manual Lymph Drainage, by Dr. Vodder

Pain Erasure, by Bonnie Prudden

Sports Massage, by Jack Meagher & Pat Boughton

Whole Body Healing, published by Prevention Magazine

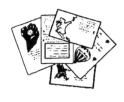

GREETING CARDS
FOR MASSAGE PROFESSIONALS

All Occasion Cards:
Maryann Capó, Ten Plus Ten
469 Hawkins Ave., Suite 202
Lake Ronkonkoma, NY 11779
(See order form on last page)

Holiday Only:
Health Management Group
3742 Arelia Drive North
Delray Beach, FL 33445
(407) 393-1139

MASSAGE MAGAZINES

The Bodywork Entrepreneur
584 Castro Street, Suite 373
San Francisco, CA 94114

The Florida State Massage Message
PO Box 1983
Sarasota, FL 34230

Massage Magazine
PO Box 1389
Kailua-Kona, HI 96745

The Massage Therapy Journal (AMTA)
1130 W. North Shore Avenue
Chicago, IL 60626

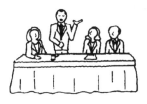

MASSAGE ORGANIZATIONS

Alliance of Massage Therapists
c/o Swedish Institute
226 West 26th Street
New York, NY 10001
(212) 840-7788

American International Reiki Association
2210 Wilshire Blvd. Suite 831
Santa Monica, CA 90403
(214) 788-1821

American Massage Therapy Association, Inc.
1130 W. North Shore Avenue
Chicago, IL 60626
(312) 761-AMTA

The American Polarity Therapy Association
PO Box 44154
Somerville, MA   02144
(617) 776-6696

California Health Practitioners Association
PO Box 90875
San Diego, CA   92109
(619) 234-5662

Florida State Massage Therapists Association
5473 66th Street North
St. Petersburg, FL   33709
(813)541-2666

International Sports Massage Federation
120 East 18th Street
Costa Mesa, CA   92627
(714)642-0735

International Association of Infant Massage Instructors
PO Box 16103
Portland, OR   97216
(503) 253-9977

New York State Society of Medical Massage Therapists
PO Box 826
Glenwood Landing, NY   11547
(516) 697-7668

Northwest Massage Practitioners Association
1605 12th Avenue #27
Seattle, WA   98122
(206) 324-1491

On-Site Massage Association
584 Castro Street Suite 373
San Francisco, CA 94114-2588
(415) 621-6817

The Rolf® Institute
PO Box 1868
Boulder, CO 80306
(303) 449-5903

Shiatsu Practitioners Association
2309 Main Street
Santa Monica, CA 90405
(213) 396-4877

Trager® Institute
10 Old Mill
Mill Valley, CA 94941
(415) 388-2688

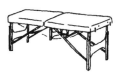 **MASSAGE TABLES AND CHAIRS**

Living Earth Crafts
600 East Todd Road
Santa Rose, CA 95407
1-800-358-8292
Portable Tote Table
High-Touch Chair
Massage Mate Desk Top System

Oakworks, Inc.
427 South Main Street
Shrewsbury, PA   17361
1-800-558-8850
Shelved tables
The Portal (Massage Chair)

Pisces Productions
PO Box 208
Cotati, CA   94928
1-800-TABLE-33
Portable table with Adjustable Headrest
The Dolphin Massage Chair

Stacey-Built Systems
PO Box 1032
Clinton, NC   28328
1-800-356-8426
Backsaver Table, with electric lift control

Touch America
PO Box 1304
Hillsborough, NC   27278
1-800-678-6824
Shelved table
The Body Chair

Ultra-Light, Inc.
16 Dickinson Avenue
Toms River, NJ   08753
1-800-999-1971
The Ultra-Light, lightest table on the market

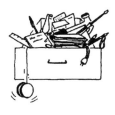 MISCELLANEOUS

Anatomical Charts Co.
8221 North Kimball
Skokie, IL 60076
1-800-621-7500

Bongers — wholesale
Body Tools
15829 Haynes Street
Van Nuys, CA 91406

Bongers — retail
Maryann Capó
469 Hawkins Avenue Suite 202
Lake Ronkonkoma, NY 11779
(516) 585-5691
(see order form on last page of this book)

Safeguard Business Systems
455 Maryland Drive
PO Box 7501
Fort Washington, PA 19034
1-800-523-2422
Long Island, NY, Distributor:
Bill Thorpe
PO Box 203
Kings Park, NY 11754
(516) 447-9451

Split Skirts
Haband for Her
Haband Distribution Center
Peckville, PA 18452-2016
(201) 942-1010
Colors: Cream, Rose, Marine, Chambray Blue, Wheat

Stressdots
Maryann Capó
469 Hawkins Avenue
Lake Ronkonkoma, NY 11779
(516) 585-5691
(see order form on last page of this book)

Temporary Tenant Network
TTN (Newsletter)
PO Box 130
Jefferson Valley, NY 10535

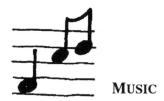 MUSIC

Environmental Tapes
Syntonic Research, Inc.
175 5th Avenue
New York, NY 10010
Slow Ocean
Sailboat
Caribbean Lagoon

Mood Tapes
Gateway Recordings
Distributed by Gemcom, Inc.
PO Box 5087
FDR Station
New York, NY 10022
(Free catalog to Dept. M)
Mountain Retreat
Backyard Stream
Tropical Rain Forest

Solitudes Tapes
Moss Music Group, Inc.
48 West 38th Street
New York, NY 10018
Sailing to a Hidden Cove/Hiking Over the Highlands
By Canoe to Loon Lake/Dawn by a Gentle Stream

Other Tapes
Mike Rowland
Distributed by Music Design, Inc.
207 East Buffalo
Milwaukee, WI 53202
Fairy Ring

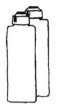 **OILS**

Biotone
3536 Adams Avenue
San Diego, CA 92116
1-800-445-6457

Soothing Touch
1919 Burnside Avenue
Los Angeles, CA 90016
(213) 939-6400

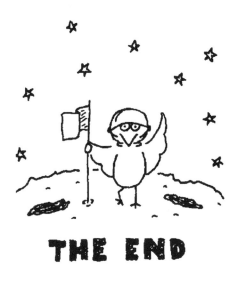

THE END

Notes:

ORDER FORM

ITEM	COST EA.	QTY	TOTAL
The Business of Massage A Manual for Students and Professionals	$18.95		
Bongers *(wrapped singly, with instructional booklet included)*	6.75		
Stickers *(oval gold foil w. black lettering: "It's Great to be Kneaded"), 100 stickers per strip*	3.75		
Bumper Sticker *(white "It's Great to be Kneaded" on RED___ or BLUE___ removable vinyl - check one)*	2.00		
Stressdots *(strip of 10 dots)*	3.50		
Stressdots *(10 dots w. booklet on recognizing stress, simple relaxation techniques, and history of stressdots)*	6.50		
In-Touch Greeting Cards *(total from other side)*			
Processing and Handling			1.00
N.Y. residents please add 8% Sales Tax			
Please allow three to four weeks for delivery	**TOTAL**		

Complete mailing address on opposite side, and send with check or money order (U.S. funds) to:
**Ten Plus Ten, 469 Hawkins Ave. Suite 202
Lk. Ronkonkoma, NY 11779**

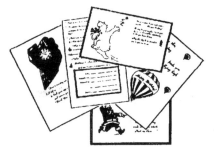

Original Greeting Cards...

Birthday, Discounts, Christmas...

The most effective way to keep your client file active and current is to "Keep In Touch"

Pack of 12 cards - $5 a set

CARD	QTY	TOTAL
0100 Birthday - Balloon		
0101 Birthday - Bear		
0200 Christmas - Santa		
0201 Christmas - Tree		
0300 Gift Certificate		
0301 10% Discount - Time Running Out		
TOTAL		**$**

- -

Your Mailing Address

Name_____

Street_____

City _____ **St** _____ **Zip** _____

Daytime Phone_____

ORDER FORM

ITEM	COST EA.	QTY	TOTAL
The Business of Massage A Manual for Students and Professionals	$18.95		
Bongers *(wrapped singly, with instruction-al booklet included)*	6.75		
Stickers *(oval gold foil w. black lettering: "It's Great to be Kneaded"), 100 stickers per strip*	3.75		
Bumper Sticker *(white "It's Great to be Kneaded" on RED___ or BLUE___ removable vinyl - check one)*	2.00		
Stressdots *(strip of 10 dots)*	3.50		
Stressdots *(10 dots w. booklet on recogniz-ing stress, simple relaxation tech-niques, and history of stressdots)*	6.50		
In-Touch Greeting Cards *(total from other side)*			
Processing and Handling			1.00
N.Y. residents please add 8% Sales Tax			
Please allow three to four weeks for delivery	**TOTAL**		

Complete mailing address on opposite side, and send with check or money order (U.S. funds) to:
**Ten Plus Ten, 469 Hawkins Ave. Suite 202
Lk. Ronkonkoma, NY 11779**

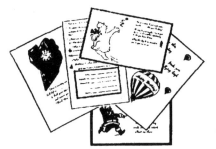

Original Greeting Cards...

Birthday, Discounts, Christmas...

The most effective way to keep your client file active and current is to "Keep In Touch"

Pack of 12 cards - $5 a set

CARD	QTY	TOTAL
0100 Birthday - Balloon		
0101 Birthday - Bear		
0200 Christmas - Santa		
0201 Christmas - Tree		
0300 Gift Certificate		
0301 10% Discount - Time Running Out		
	TOTAL	$

Your Mailing Address

Name_____

Street_____

City _____ **St** _____ **Zip** _____

Daytime Phone_____